Contents

Foreword

As a result of devolution, we are already witnessing variation between the health services of the four home nations. As time passes, divergence in relation to the structure and function in primary and community care will inevitably increase. However, employment law continues and is likely to continue as a reserved power with legislation being the responsibility of Westminster. The need for the health service and the independent employing contractors, particularly general medical practitioners, to promote and participate in good employment practice safely within the law is essential. The old adage 'prevention is better than cure' is, as always, pertinent. Good employment practice will undoubtedly be a vital element in fostering and maintaining a positive motivated workforce with resultant gains to the quality of patient care.

Principal general practitioners have defined responsibilities as employers. Although much day-to-day management is delegated to our management staff, it is crucial that we are not only knowledgeable but also actively support and enact exemplary employment as well as clinical practice. Also, in England on 1 April 2000, the first in an initial wave of 17 primary care trusts began work as commissioners and providers of primary healthcare services. One of the criteria for approval of Trust status was a commitment to a human resources strategy. Central to this requirement is the recognition that those primary care groups which have successfully applied for Trust status have moved from employing a chief executive and a few support staff to an organisation employing up to 500 people including a wide range of health professionals, some of them based in hospitals.

So, whether a Trust chair or chief executive, an established principal, a young principal or a general practitioner in training, the essentials of managing people legally and fairly in a multi-disciplinary environment is key to the success of the health service of our nation, and this book is essential reading for all those involved in employment at all levels in primary care. It provides a clear definition of good practice together with a succinct update with regard to current employment legislation. It is peppered with real-life examples which bring theory into reality within the context of practice-based primary care.

For practice managers, as well as being an excellent reference, it provides a catalyst to revisit a number of issues within the practice. It highlights the need for the development of important policy statements as a matter of good organisational governance. In particular, from my recent experience supporting two managers preparing for Fellowship by Assessment of the Institute of Healthcare Management (IHM), I know that this text will be a core resource in supporting Fellowship of the IHM in the future.

Colin M Hunter OBE MB ChB DRCOG FRCGP FRCP (Edinburgh)
General Practitioner, Aberdeen
National Co-ordinator for Primary Care
Postgraduate Medical & Dental Education for Scotland
October 2000

About the authors

Hilary Haman is a Fellow of the Chartered Institute of Personnel and Development and a Member of the Institute of Healthcare Management.

She has over 20 years' experience in personnel management, including running human resource departments in both the public and private sectors. Hilary first became professionally involved in primary healthcare in 1986 when she joined the Royal College of General Practitioners in London as head of personnel.

Since 1990 she has worked as an independent management consultant, mainly in general practice, although she has other clients in the private, public and voluntary sectors. Her work encompasses providing advice on personnel issues, including the application of employment law, designing and running management development courses and, with Sally Irvine as Haman and Irvine Associates, undertaking organisational reviews of individual practices and developing management tools for general practice.

She writes extensively on management and personnel issues within primary care and lives in Cardiff with her husband and son.

Sally Irvine was made an Honorary Fellow of the Royal College of General Practitioners in 1995, a Fellow of the Association of Managers in General Practice in the same year and is a Member of the Institute of Healthcare Management.

She has over 15 years' experience of working in and with many aspects of healthcare delivery. She was the general administrator of the RCGP from 1984 to 1994, and was president of the AMGP from 1990 to 1994. She chaired Newcastle City Health NHS Trust, which delivered community, mental health and rehabilitative care in the north-east of England, from its inception in 1993 to 1999. Currently she is appointed a lay member of the General Dental Council and a hospital manager under the Mental Health Act. Her most recent appointments are as an arbitrator for the Advisory and Conciliation and Arbitration Service (ACAS), a member of the Newcastle Common Purpose Advisory Board and a trustee of Total Learning Challenge.

In recent years Sally has concentrated on her work as a professional practice consultant in primary care. She has published many texts on organisational and development issues within primary care and writes regularly for the medical press.

Introduction

Successful managers today have to ask themselves 'Am I learning as fast as the world is changing?' This book is one tool in that learning process. It provides a guide through the employment journey, starting with the recruitment and selection of staff, the ways of offering appropriate terms and conditions of employment and later training and promotion opportunities. During this journey managers have to establish and maintain a relationship of trust, respect and confidence with staff and deal with issues such as pregnancy and parenting, relationships between colleagues and grievances, both overt and covert. The journey ends with the person leaving the organisation either through resignation or retirement or, more problematically, through redundancy or some other form of dismissal.

In this journey the emphasis is clearly on employed staff, but the inter-relationships and interdependencies involved, and the skills and attitudes described, are as relevant for partnerships and the different primary care groupings of England, Wales and Scotland as they are for the more conventional manager/subordinate relationships.

This book is based on the premise that all organisations depend for their success on the ability of the people who work within them to give of their best to each other. In general practice particularly, effective networking between people from different professions and with different skills and responsibilities depends on an understanding of, and sensitivity to, each other's needs, motivations and abilities. Primary care, however it develops, will always be a 'people-dependent' service. The immediate needs of those people – be they doctors, nurses, members or administrators of the different primary care boards, practice administrative or reception staff – must be satisfied. At the same time, their potential needs have to be developed to ensure that, at all times, patient care is being provided to the optimum level by a happy, fulfilled and stimulated team.

Over the past 20 years the face of primary care has changed beyond all recognition. The prominence given to general practice within a primary care-led National Health Service (NHS) by the Conservative government through the 1980s and 1990s and continued by the Labour government elected in 1997, continues into the 21st century. The programme of change that the present government has introduced was first outlined at the end of 1997 in three White Papers (Department of Health 1997, 1998a,b). It involved restructuring NHS trusts (in Scotland and Wales in particular their numbers have been substantially reduced), a more strategic role for health authorities and radical changes to primary care. This programme of change accelerates the need for both individual practices and the boards of primary care groups (England), local health groups (Wales) and local healthcare co-operatives (Scotland) to change their approach to the management of people. For simplification, all three types of group will be referred to as primary care groups (PCGs). The government, in its White Papers, made clear that good human resource management is vital to its efforts to modernise the NHS and specified staff commitment and involvement as being crucial to the delivery of high-quality patient care.

The changes to primary healthcare and its management have given doctors the opportunity to opt for a role in primary care other than as a traditional practice partner. For example, there has been an increase in the number of practice assistants and doctors on the Doctor Retainer Schemes, the introduction of salaried general practitioners to primary care and the appointment of general practitioners to PCGs. The personnel management demands made on primary care managers, both clinical and non-clinical, are extremely complex, particularly for PCGs and future primary care trusts (PCTs), as the employment environment in which such boards operate is still ambiguous and unclear.

There are a number of other external factors that have also come into play:

- accountability and health medicine
- social change
- new employment legislation
- the sociological and economic climate
- performance management.

Accountability and health medicine

One of the most fundamental changes affecting personnel management and planning in primary care has been the expectation of accountability, by health professions and institutions, to the public, the government and the medical profession itself.

The National Institute for Clinical Excellence (NICE) is intended to provide a framework of national guidelines against which health service performance may be measured in due course. The Commission for Health Improvement (CHI) has powers to scrutinise health institutions and call them to account managerially. In Scotland, these functions are undertaken by the Scottish Intercollegiate Guidelines Network (SIGN) and the Clinical Standards Board, respectively. The schemes for revalidation under the umbrella of the General Medical Council (GMC) and implemented by the individual royal medical colleges will demand a level of professional accountability hitherto lacking. The introduction of clinical governance requires PCGs, trusts and general practice to put in place arrangements to ensure that quality is guaranteed. Continuing professional development (CPD) has brought to the fore the need for professionally managed programmes of training, education and development for all members of the primary care team. The different methods the profession is now being encouraged to adopt in identifying educational needs have raised the profile of performance management, extending appraisal from managers appraising staff to peer appraisal in the practice and postgraduate setting (Van Zwanenberg and Harrison 2000). The practice of undertaking courses or programmes of training on whim or interest is being replaced by a far more structured and strategic process of educational plans for the whole practice through professional practice development plans (PPDPs) and, linked with these, personal development plans (PDPs).

Social change

In addition to the fundamental changes made in the clinical, organisational, educational and quality assurance demands of primary care, there have been profound changes in employment legislation introduced by the government and the European Union (EU) of which all employers need to be aware. In the recent past, general practices were staffed by personnel who, in the main, worked part time, whose personal loyalty to the practice was high but whose knowledge, awareness and interest in legal rights of employment were low. This is in contrast with other sectors of the UK where the numbers of people using employment tribunals to resolve issues of unfair dismissal and breaches of contracts of employment was high and which continues to rise.

Primary care has been relatively successful in avoiding litigation, only paying lip service to many areas of employee rights and developments and, in the process, missing opportunities to motivate, retain and develop staff successfully. For example, a written practice equal opportunities policy in which the entire team is trained is still a rarity in general practice, and such developments continue to be seen by many as superfluous to the reality of everyday working life.

These legislative and sociological changes are now coupled with an economic environment that has the lowest inflation rate for 36 years and the lowest unemployment rate for 20 years. Competition for skilled personnel and the ability to retain them will assume a much greater importance in organisational effectiveness and success.

New employment legislation

Employment legislation in the UK is complex and, through case law, often contradictory. For example, the details of maternity rights and their application taxes even the most skilled of personnel managers. The definitions of disability under the 1995 Disability Discrimination Act continue to be regularly challenged through employment tribunals.

From 1 June 1999 employees' rights in seeking legal redress to claims of unfair dismissal have been strengthened and, in December 1999, individual employees gained parental and domestic leave rights. The year 2000 saw changes to maternity rights and, perhaps the most significant change of all, trade union recognition (Department of Trade and Industry 1999). Managers in primary care are entering an industrial relations environment of which most have little knowledge and even less experience.

This new arena will have a direct and indirect impact on individual relations between employees, relations between employees and management, and direct financial implications in the terms and conditions of employment. A new equality is emerging, shifting some of the power from employers to employees and their representatives. PCGs and individual practices must be part of this new world.

The propensity for litigation experienced in the medical world has been mirrored and exceeded by that in the world of industrial relations. So these legislative changes are taking place in a more litigious environment. The diminishing of trade union power and the cycle of economic boom and bust of the 1980s have made people, as individuals, more self-reliant and willing to take employers to court. For example, the number of individual conciliation cases in which the Advisory and Conciliation and Arbitration Service (ACAS) has been involved rose by 43% between 1994 and 1998, from 79 332 to 113 636 (ACAS 1998).

The sociological and economic climate

The country we now live in has been transformed from the UK of the 1970s. Economically we have moved away from a manufacturing to a service-based economy – people are buying the gardener rather than the lawnmower! There is no longer an expectation that one job will see an employee throughout his or her life and young people now expect to be helped to cross bridges rather than climb ladders. Along with this is an expectation that employers will provide the development of employees, even if this means that such development enables them to leave the organisation. Thirty-five is no longer young and 60 is no longer old. The general practice of today has people within it who are better educated, more sophisticated and more aware of their rights. They also have higher expectations of their employers and managers who assume that their own developmental needs will be addressed. Indeed this commitment by employers to staff and professional development was made explicit by the Department of Health in its definition of CPD:

> ... a process of lifelong learning for all individuals and teams which meets the needs of patients and delivers the health outcomes and healthcare priorities of the NHS and which enables professionals to expand and fulfil their potential. (DoH 1998c)

With high levels of employment, the current economic situation will lead to even greater competition between employers for skilled and committed staff and therefore the retention of effective employees will assume a greater importance.

Now is the time for individual managers within primary care organisations to prepare themselves for the new work environment. It should enable them to gain the confidence needed to exploit these changes to the benefit of primary care rather than see them as threats to the individual power bases occupied by individual doctors and general practice partnerships. Managers in primary care need to be at least as skilled in managing people as they are in managing money.

Performance management

The Chartered Institute of Personnel and Development (CIPD) in its paper *Employment Relations into the 21st Century* (CIPD 1997) anticipates the changes managers of people will need to face in this new century. Experienced personnel practitioners have always known that the way people are managed is the key factor in organisational success. Most employers want the following from their staff:

- willingness to change
- business orientation
- a sense of individual responsibility
- strong teamworking
- the use of initiative
- a commitment to organisational objectives, processes and programmes
- the giving of discretionary effort – a willing contribution
- continuous learning.

The skill of management is to help staff fulfil these expectations while meeting the employee's needs, which, from studying current research and the observations of practitioners, appear to be:

- **reward**, the fairness of the process within which it is determined and the outcome in relation to other employees
- **job satisfaction** in relation to the intrinsic interest of the job and its design
- **skill development and technology upgrading**, adding significantly to a sense of self-worth
- **relationships with managers**, directly and in cross-functional structures
- **wellbeing** – a sense of employment security with the same or another employer, involvement and trust that management decisions are being taken in ways which reflect, as far as possible, the best interests of employees (Guest and Conway 1997).

The CIPD (1997) has identified two areas which require attention in employment relations in the 21st century:

> ... making sure that people management and development practices in individual organisations add up to a coherent system designed to achieve what the organisation wants ... and thinking through the feedback routes by which the views of employees are gathered together – listening to the voice of employees.

If primary healthcare is to fulfil the ambition of providing consistent, high-quality care by individuals and teams who are motivated, supportive and skilled, it will be imperative that managers (including partners in practice and doctors on primary care boards) move from reactive activities to planned, proactive and sophisticated styles, methods and programmes of management with the views of individuals and teams taking centre stage.

1
Entry into employment

Successful recruitment is a key managerial task, the importance of which is often underestimated. Employing organisations are social institutions where we fulfil both formal and informal roles and functions. The standard of work performed by an organisation's personnel is the single major factor which differentiates the excellent from the merely good business, and the good from the mediocre (Hunt 1990). Employers therefore need to ensure that when people enter into employment, the process that is undertaken is thorough and robust and ensures that the right people are in the right place doing the right job at the right time.

The advantages of a good recruitment process are set out in Box 1.1.

Box 1.1: Advantages of good recruitment procedures

Good recruitment procedures ensure that:

- a positive image of the organisation is given to all candidates including those who are unsuccessful and who may be customers, clients or patients, or indeed future employees
- applicants have an accurate understanding of the organisation and what will be expected of them
- the risk of a poor selection decision is reduced
- the risk of litigation is reduced, but if it does arise the procedure will provide a sound defence for the organisation

General practice surgeries and medical centres are people-based organisations. The introduction of the different PCGs in

England, Wales and Scotland has both added to the complexity of employment relationships in primary care and emphasised the need for great care in carrying out this basic responsibility of managers everywhere. However, as with many other organisations, recruitment in primary care is often undertaken in a haphazard manner with the quality and, frequently, the procedural rigour of the task being determined by whoever is undertaking it. This can result in different standards in the same organisation and applicants having different recruitment experiences. This is a concern, as the recruitment process is often the first experience a potential employee has of an organisation.

When someone applies for a vacancy, neither the employer nor the applicant knows with any certainty how long the relationship will last. With the exception of staff on fixed-term contracts, the length of the employment relationship can range from a few days to many years. However long or short it is, the investment by both parties in the relationship is significant. For the employer it represents a considerable investment in money, time, space and equipment, based on a trust that the employee will work well and honestly. For the employee it represents an investment of time, professional skills and knowledge, together with the major step of placing trust in a particular employer that they will deliver security of employment and career development. Depending on the status and importance of the job, both parties will have considerable expectations of the other. Unfortunately this means many employment relationships are characterised by disappointment. Employers can be disappointed with the level of productivity of the employee in return for the high level of payment made, and the employee can be disappointed in the remuneration and benefits given for all the work that he or she does.

It is vital therefore that, before a contract of employment is offered and accepted, these expectations are clarified and tested. This testing is the exercise that underpins and is the main objective of the recruitment and selection process. It is a two-way process and in these days of better-educated people with higher expectations, the applicant will expect as much of the employer as the employer does of the applicant.

Moreover, the entry into employment is also one of the most vulnerable activities for employers in terms of litigation for illegal discrimination (Chapter 3 addresses the area of illegal discrimination in more detail). It is a management activity that is open to subjective feelings and hastily made decisions. There is now a considerable body of statute and case law that has to be observed throughout the whole process. It is vital therefore that all practices and primary care boards, regardless of size and resources, develop a recruitment procedure that is known to all staff and in which all those carrying it out are trained. Following a well-thought through procedure ensures that standards and recruitment systems are fair, consistent and valid, and that equal opportunity is an integral part of the process.

The main components of an effective recruitment procedure are set out in Box 1.2.

Box 1.2: Components of a recruitment procedure

- developing the documentation, namely a job description and personal specification
- designing and placing the advertisement(s)
- administering applications
- selecting for interview
- establishing interviewing principles and practice
- selecting the successful candidate
- making the appointment

This chapter addresses:

- the ways of reducing the risks of making bad appointments by applying a well-thought out and skilful recruitment and selection procedure
- the role such a procedure plays in the wider management of an organisation

- the induction of new colleagues
- the more subtle areas of the contract of employment
- the legislation involved in recruiting and selecting.

First steps: is there a vacancy?

When someone is leaving, an opportunity arises to gain valuable information, not only about the job the person is leaving but also about the organisation itself. This information is gleaned through talking to the person who is leaving or conducting what is called an 'exit interview'. Honest responses are required to get the best out of such a process, and therefore this discussion is often best conducted in confidence by someone other than the person's line manager. After all, they may have been one of the reasons for the resignation in the first place. Similarly, it is important to make it clear to the person who is leaving that the employer has a genuine desire to learn what the organisation is like for those who work within it.

It is also a good idea to conduct this interview after references have been sent to the person's new employer, if this is a relevant factor, as when people leave an organisation they are sometimes anxious about the references their current employer will give. This consideration may colour the frankness with which they reflect on their experience of the organisation.

The exit interview may well identify tasks that have become obsolete, especially in organisations that are changing quickly. It may also reveal ways of distributing the work to other staff, in which case the person leaving need not be replaced. Whatever the outcome, it is important to conduct the interview sensitively and carefully, however informally, and for the interviewer to remain — and be seen to remain — impartial throughout.

The information gained from this discussion, together with a review of the organisation and its future plans and anticipated changes, will contribute to the decision whether or not to fill the vacancy and the details of the vacancy.

Example 1.1

When a practice secretary left after six years' service, she agreed to talk to the executive partner, to give him her views on the post she was vacating. She was pleased to have the chance to get off her chest some of the concerns she had been harbouring for some time about whether there was a real job for a secretary. She wondered whether a dedicated medical secretary was now needed, as the practice was fully computerised. She confessed that she had felt rather like a dogsbody in the last few years. She had been given some fairly menial tasks to fill her time. She had thought that the only reason she had not been made redundant was due to the partners' concerns for the fact that she was a single mother struggling to bring up her two daughters.

Now she was leaving she thought the practice should review her job. The partner was grateful to have this clear steer, and relieved that they could consider replacing the secretary with a more generally qualified administrator, without everyone feeling uncomfortable.

The job description and personal specification

Once clear about the type of vacancy, preparatory work needs to be done on two important documents – the job description and the personal specification. These are crucial in ensuring that as objective an assessment as possible is used in selecting the right candidate.

The job description describes the main duties and responsibilities of the vacancy. The personal specification describes the type of person needed to undertake those duties and responsibilities. It is important not to confuse the two, and to write the former before the latter. It is easy to merge them and thus immediately start imagining the type of person to employ **before** a complete and objective analysis and description of the post has taken place.

Each organisation and each job differs so there is no set format to a job description. However, for it to be meaningful and help in successful recruitment there are a number of basic ingredients. These are set out in Box 1.3.

Box 1.3: Basic ingredients of a job description

- the job title
- the main terms of reference
- the person to whom the person will be accountable
- an indication of those with whom the job holder will work
- the main responsibilities and duties of the post, including responsibilities for other staff, materials and money

The list of main responsibilities needs to be fleshed out into some form of meaningful description and time needs to be spent on identifying a set of competencies that are needed to do the job.

Once these have been identified, the work can start on producing the second crucial document – the personal specification. This translates the job description into a profile of the person required to do the job. This profile is expressed in terms of:

- the skills, knowledge, aptitude and experience needed
- the qualifications necessary to do the job unless recruitment is undertaken on the future potential of the candidate, for instance when someone newly qualified is considered
- personal qualities relevant to the job, such as genuine commitment to the health service/patient care or the ability to work as part of a team.

The particular factors identified under each of the above headings need to be separated into those that are prerequisites to do the job at the required level immediately, known as 'essential' factors, and those factors that would help the person do the job but which are only 'desirable'.

Advertising the post

The job description and personal specification together should help draw up the advertisement. In particular, the advertisement should contain enough of the 'essential' factors to attract eligible candidates and deter unqualified ones. Box 1.4 sets out the elements needed to ensure that advertisements are effective and free from bias.

Box 1.4: Elements of an advertisement

- the requirements of the job
- the essential and some desirable criteria of applicants
- the activities and working practices of the organisation
- the location of the vacancy
- the reward package
- contract length, if relevant
- application procedure and closing date for applications

It is important both morally and legally to ensure that no sections of the community are discouraged from applying by the way advertisements are worded or visually presented. The following is an example of unacceptable wording:

> We are seeking a receptionist who is willing to work longer hours at short notice and able to act as a chaperone to female patients when they are being examined by our male doctors. The job would suit a local person who has previous experience of working with the public.

The above extract from an advertisement discourages people from outside the immediate locality (and this could be racially discriminatory) and those who have personal commitments which would prevent them from undertaking overtime at short notice. This latter category would include people with young families and is, therefore, in contravention of the Sex

Discrimination Act. The advert also implies, through reference to chaperone duties, that females only should apply. Again this is in contravention of the Sex Discrimination Act unless it comes under a Genuine Occupational Qualification (see Chapter 3).

Also, advertisements should not make misleading claims. There is no law to prevent discriminating on grounds of age, except where it includes indirect sex or race discrimination. However the government has produced a code on age discrimination (Department of Education and Employment 1999b) and it is expected that legislation will follow if employers fail to follow the code and continue to implement age barriers in recruitment and employment. It is advisable, therefore, to ensure that no age barriers or age-related criteria of any description are used. The following is an example of unacceptable wording:

> We are seeking a young, dynamic manager with at least 7 years' managerial experience and with the physical and mental stamina to handle this demanding executive post.

The above extract from an advertisement could be seen to discourage people with a disability and also exclude a large proportion of female managers, many of whom, due to career breaks for family reasons, will not have gained seven years' experience while still 'young'. Thus it constitutes indirect sex discrimination, which is discussed more fully in Chapter 3. In addition, the advert also runs counter to the government's voluntary code to eliminate discrimination on the grounds of age. A more acceptable alternative wording would be as follows:

> We are seeking a manager with at least 7 years' managerial experience who has the commitment and drive to undertake this demanding executive post.

Applications

When people respond to a job advertisement and request an application form, they should be given the name of the person they can contact to confirm that their application has been received. Prompt acknowledgement presents a positive image of the organisation. Applicants should also be advised (usually on the application form or in the information given to applicants prior to pre-selection screening) that data entered on application forms will be kept confidential by the organisation in accordance with the Data Protection Acts 1984 and 1998. The latter Act relates to manual, paper-based information collected on or after 28 October 1998. Applicants should be confident that all applications are treated confidentially and only circulated to those involved in the recruitment process. The first task is to screen them against the personal specification. This is where the preparation of this document reaps huge benefits in terms of objectivity and time. Applicants who do not meet the essential criteria can safely be rejected at this point. This is effectively a system of shortlisting for interview that is objective and moreover ensures that lawful criteria are being used in the selection process. This minimises the risks of prejudice and subjectivity.

Interviewing applicants

Why interview?

The purposes of a recruitment interview are:

- for the organisation to get as much information as possible about the candidate in order to make a judgement of their suitability for the job
- similarly for candidates to receive sufficient information in order to make a judgement about the job on offer
- for both parties to explore the potential match between the individual and the organisation.

Although there are many forms of selecting people for posts, including assessment centres and psychometric tests, nothing can replace the interview as the main method of selecting staff. Those who are most closely concerned with the vacancy can explore with an applicant in a face-to-face situation the 'fit' between the person and the organisation, their skills and experience, and the needs of the post.

Preparing for the interview

Preparation is the key to successful interviewing. Preparation includes the practicalities of giving adequate notice of the interview, directions on how to get to the interview and keeping to appointment times. These are all important in this public relations exercise. In addition, such information and behaviour will help the interviewee to relax and thus give the best of himself or herself. It is of no benefit to anyone to exacerbate the natural anxiety that people feel at interviews through poor communications and an unfriendly environment. Relaxing candidates is essential if authentic information is to be gleaned and 'stress' interviews therefore are not usually an effective method of selection. A relaxed and informal style of questioning and allowing the candidate to discuss responses in detail all help in this aim.

Decisions need to be made as to who will interview. Interview panels of more than four people may daunt interviewees. Moreover, they may mean there is insufficient time for interviewers to develop in-depth questions to probe candidates. A chair should be appointed and he or she should allocate the areas to be explored. All, and particularly the chair, should be trained in recruitment interviewing techniques. Each interviewer should write down the opening and follow-up questions in his or her area of questioning. All questions should relate to the qualities sought as identified on the personal specification and should not under any circumstances stray into areas of illegal discrimination (see Chapter 3). Box 1.5 gives some simple dos and don'ts for effective interviews.

Box 1.5: Dos and don'ts of effective interviews

Do	Don't
plan the interview	start the interview unprepared
establish an easy and informal relationship	plunge too quickly into demanding questions
encourage the candidate to talk	ask leading questions
cover the ground as planned	jump to conclusions on inadequate evidence
probe where necessary	pay too much attention to isolated strengths or weaknesses
analyse career and interests to reveal strengths and weaknesses, patterns of behaviour	allow the candidate to gloss over important facts
maintain control over the direction and time taken by the interview	talk too much

Interview procedure

To help the interview, you should use a simple assessment form to record each candidate's response. Box 1.6 gives an example of such a form and Box 1.7 sets out the advantages of using such an assessment form.

Part of the training of interviewers, referred to above, needs to ensure that all are aware that notes made at interview may be revealed to an employment tribunal should a disgruntled applicant decide to sue. In addition, under the new Data Protection Act, the applicant may request direct access to interview records.

At the end of the interview, candidates should be informed of the timescale of the appointment and how they will be informed of the result. This information should err on the side of generosity, as decisions can take longer than first anticipated and every effort should be made to comply with the timescales

Box 1.6: Interview assessment sheet

Vacancy: . . . . Interviewers: . . . . Date: . . . .

Candidate: . . . . Time in: . . . .

Time out: . . . .

Factor	Criteria						Comments
		Essential			Desirable		
		Not met	Partially	Met	Not met	Partially	Met	

Box 1.7: Advantages of using an assessment form

- to minimise the problem of interviewers confusing the candidates
- to ensure a record is being maintained throughout the interview
- to help identify discrepancies which can be explored later in the interview
- to accord with the discrimination codes of practice (see Chapter 3) on the elimination of sex, race and disability discrimination in employment
- to help ensure that assessments made about a candidate are objective

given. Candidates should always be alerted to the possibility of any delays, and be notified if any unforeseen ones arise.

Selecting the successful candidate

Selecting the successful candidate should be done only after all candidates have been interviewed and each has been assessed in relation to the job description and personal specification. The interview assessment form (see Box 1.6) is extremely useful at this point in the process. It provides an objective record of the candidate's history and interview performance against which the personal specification is compared. Candidates should be identified as suitable or not suitable for the job under discussion on their own merits. The temptation, at this point, to compare candidates with each other must be resisted. Only if there are two or more who are deemed fit for the job should they be compared with each other. Otherwise the panel may fall into the trap of appointing the best of a bad or mediocre bunch.

At this point it is worth mentioning a much-neglected area in primary healthcare recruitment of both medical and non-medical personnel, and that is checking out the honesty of candidates.

Research shows that a third of companies do not check the qualifications of candidates despite a quarter of firms reporting that poor performance is one of the main reasons for staff losses

(Prickett 1998). Another report from the Association of Search and Selection Consultants found that a quarter of all curriculum vitaes (CVs) contained lies (Prickett 1998).

Even though checking people's credentials does cost time and money, an organisation need only make one major mistake to spend the same resources on clearing up the mess afterwards. It is worth bearing in mind the unpleasant fact that in 1998 two-thirds of companies in the Top 1000 companies published by *The Times* had been victims of financial fraud in the previous 12 months, and that in 84% of cases the fraud had been perpetrated by employees (Midgley 1999).

A CV containing inaccuracies or deliberate frauds can lead to dangerous malpractice in cases where the qualifications set out in the CV confirm vital skills. The types of professional and range of staff, including salaried GPs, now being employed in primary care, has increased. A recruitment procedure that does not contain a process for authenticating CVs may lead to problems in the future, including legal liability. The competitive nature of today's job market means that more and more recruits are being tempted to embellish, if not falsify, their CVs.

The key elements involved in such an effective vetting process are set out in Box 1.8. The desirable way forward, however, is to prevent it happening, and one of the most important preventative measures is to warn candidates on the application form or in any letters sent to them that the employer reserves the right to check an individual's record with *all* former employers. It is also important to ensure that applicants are asked to state in writing their reasons for leaving past employers. Applicants should be asked to bring original certificates to interviews, particularly degree and professional qualifications; photocopies are too easy to forge. Finally, as a last resort on the prevention front, all applicants should be asked to sign their completed application forms as being true. If later they are found to have lied, the employee may be dismissed as the relationship of trust and confidence between employee and employer (described in Chapter 2) has been breached.

Box 1.8: Vetting application forms

- scrutinise application forms, note down any gaps and make intelligent cross-connections rather than merely performing mechanical checks, e.g. comparing the dates of someone's schooling and university years with their date of birth
- a person's employment history should contain months and not just the years they were employed; it is not difficult to disguise a year's absence when just noting down years of employment
- follow up references – talk to referees and do not rely wholly on what is written down
- test critical skills, such as languages or knowledge of computer programs rather than relying on the CV
- try not to become complacent and assume that if someone has had two or three previous jobs then past employers have done the checking

---

Post-interview procedures

Notifying the candidates

Writing to all unsuccessful candidates should be undertaken after the successful candidate has accepted the offer of employment. Such rejection letters should be written promptly. Some candidates may telephone or write and ask why they have been rejected. There is no legal obligation to respond. However, it is helpful for candidates to know the reasons why they have been unsuccessful – they have after all invested time and energy in applying for the post. Responses should not address candidates' personalities but should concentrate rather on the factors that the interview panel felt were strongest in the successful candidate, and on which they can build in the future.

Documentation

The recruitment and selection of staff should be carefully documented. Accurate notes and the reasons for selecting and rejecting at each stage should be maintained. One of the reasons for keeping such documentation is that in cases of alleged illegal discrimination that are brought before employment tribunals, such records form an important part of the employer's defence. Indeed, failure to have maintained such records would be viewed as a breach of the ACAS Codes of Practice in this area of employment law.

References

The post-interview procedure is not complete until references have been sought. As mentioned above, following up references is important. Many managers have become cynical about their efficacy because of the perceived dishonesty of many employers who give glowing testimonials regardless of the quality of the candidate. Such practices can be overcome through ensuring that references requested are specific and detailed in the information needed and supporting evidence required. If necessary, recruiters should not hesitate in following up with a telephone call to a referee. As far as the new Data Protection Act is concerned references are still protected from access by employees as long as the referee has stated that the reference given is private and confidential. Before revealing such references to an employee, permission needs to be obtained from the author.

Medical examinations

Prior to the Disability Discrimination Act 1995 (DDA) asking new staff to complete a medical questionnaire and/or undergo a medical examination was common practice in many organisations. However, the DDA has now made such practices questionable and they could be used at an employment tribunal to demonstrate bias on the part of the employer. It is now advisable to use medical examinations only if fitness is a key component of the ability to perform the job and it is highly unlikely that any post in primary healthcare would have such criteria.

Once the post-interview procedures have been completed and an offer of employment has been accepted, a legal relationship is formed between the successful candidate and the organisation. This is the contract of employment. It is such an important part of the process that we reserve the whole of the next chapter to define and address the formation of the contract of employment.

2
The contract of employment

The making of a contract

The last chapter discussed best practice in the recruitment and selection of employees. Once the successful candidate has been offered the job and the main terms and conditions of employment have been accepted, a contract exists between the employee and employer. It is a common misconception that a contract does not exist if no written statement has been drawn up; employees at common law are bound to their employers by individual contracts, even if there is nothing in writing. The absence of a written statement merely makes enforcing the agreed terms, or changing them, more difficult.

Nevertheless many offers are conditional, for instance upon satisfactory references or the successful completion of a probationary period. Should any of the conditional elements not be fulfilled, then the offer of employment can be withdrawn without the employer breaching a contract of employment. Example 2.1 illustrates the point.

Example 2.1

A practice was promised money by their health authority to employ an assistant GP. They went ahead and made an appointment and the doctor was sent the standard British Medical Association contract and a covering letter stating that the offer was subject to health authority

> funding. Before the assistant formally accepted the post and a month before he was due to commence, the health authority informed the practice that, due to budgetary constraints, they could not honour their promise. The practice was worried that if they withdrew the offer of employment they would be sued for breach of contract.
>
> However, they sought advice and were informed that as they had wisely placed a condition on the offer of employment, namely the availability of health authority funding, the offer could be withdrawn without fear of litigation. They were also informed that for a contract to exist there must be an unqualified acceptance of that offer. As they had yet to receive such an acceptance, no contract existed between the practice and the prospective assistant.

Contract law

Like all employers, GPs are bound by law in their employment of staff. The contract of employment is *the* basic institution of employment law. The one-to-one contract between employer and employee stands at the heart of our complex employment law, and is the means of regulating relations between employee and employer.

Many organisations design a contract with a written statement of the main terms and conditions of employment. They issue it without regularly reviewing its relevance and accuracy, either in relation to the individual and the post offered or to changes in employment law. The relevance and accuracy of these written terms become crucial if either party:

- disputes the terms and conditions of employment
- wishes to change the terms of the contract
- decides to terminate the contract of employment.

The contract of employment is comprised of five elements: written and agreed 'express' terms, implied terms, custom and practice, incorporated terms and statutory terms. These are now described.

Express terms

Employers of any size, including general practices, are required to give written statements of the main terms and conditions of employment to their staff within two months of the employee commencing employment. These main terms as specified in the Employment Rights Act 1996 are set out in Box 2.1.

Box 2.1: Minimum terms to be given to staff in writing

- the parties to the contract, i.e. the employer's and the employee's names
- the date the employment began
- continuity of employment, i.e. it is advisable to state whether or not employment with another employer, such as another practice, will count as continuous employment; a significant matter as the majority of legal rights employees enjoy are determined by length of service
- details of length of service where the employment is not permanent
- the place of work
- the address of the employer
- the title of the job the employee is employed to do
- the scale or rate of remuneration, method of calculating remuneration
- the intervals at which salary/wages are paid (monthly, weekly, etc.)
- any terms relating to hours of working including normal hours of work. Bank Holiday arrangements should also be included
- the length of notice which the employee is obliged to give and entitled to receive to terminate the contract
- the entitlement to holidays, including public holidays and holiday pay
- any terms and conditions relating to incapacity for work due to sickness or injury, including any sick pay provisions
- any terms and conditions relating to pensions and pension schemes
- details of any collective agreements which affect the employee's terms and conditions and, where the employer was not a party, by whom they were made
- details of any disciplinary rules, and the organisation's grievance procedure, including the name of the person to whom a grievance should be addressed (see Chapter 8)
- whether a pensions contracting out certificate is in force

In addition to the minimum terms outlined, employers should also include other terms of employment, which they wish to be contractually binding on both employer and employee. Examples of such additional terms include a retirement age and the right to give pay in lieu of notice. However, there will also be terms which employees should receive in writing but which the employer may not wish to make contractual. For example, annual salary increases cannot always be guaranteed. To give the practice flexibility and avoid any possibility of litigation, should staff not receive an annual increase, this term could be expressed as follows:

> Salary reviews are normally undertaken annually and any salary increases are wholly at the discretion of the partners taking into account ...

There is a golden rule in designing written statements of terms and conditions of employment, and indeed employment policies and procedures: if you think something might happen, make clear how it will be dealt with, using unambiguous wording. It is important to make clear those terms that are discretionary and therefore not contractual, as the above example of the salary increase shows. It can save a lot of time, money, emotion and adverse industrial relations if the major terms are put into the contract of employment in written form, clearly expressed.

Implied terms

There are many rights and obligations on either side that are left unexpressed and unspecified. The general rule is that a term will be implied in a contract if it is necessary to give it business efficacy or if it is so obvious that it does not need expressing.

Terms commonly implied are the employees' duties of:

- fidelity
- obedience
- working with diligence and care

and the employer's duties:

- to maintain a relationship of trust and confidence with the employee
- to provide a safe system of work and a safe working environment
- to provide wages; there is no general duty to provide work
- to act reasonably.

It is breaches of the implied, rather than the expressed terms, that often give rise to disputes that end up before employment tribunals. The following two examples demonstrate that the written terms and their interpretation are very straightforward compared with the requirement to abide by the implied terms of contracts of employment.

Example 2.2

The partners of a practice decided to merge with a neighbouring practice. They initiated and completed negotiations without telling any of their staff, who were informed of the decision by employees at the other surgery. When confronted, the partners admitted that the practices would be merging but that they had yet to decide which jobs would not be needed. It was only the skilful intervention of the senior partner of the other practice that prevented collective resignation of the staff. There could have been claims of constructive dismissal on grounds of destroying the relationship of trust and confidence and failing to act reasonably.

The same breaches are evident in Example 2.3.

Example 2.3

One of the partners in a three-partner practice had a very robust style in managing the staff of the practice. He had a fierce temper and was extremely tactless. One day, after the second occasion when the practice secretary failed to pass on a message to the other partners, he shouted at her in the reception area in front of staff and patients. He then told her to go to his room, where he proceeded to call her incompetent and useless at her job, and warned her that he would be asking the practice manager to issue her with a verbal warning.

The secretary felt humiliated and considered resigning and claiming constructive dismissal. However, she was persuaded by a colleague to use the practice's grievance procedure, following which she received a full written apology from the offending partner for his unreasonable behaviour. The partners got a commitment from him that he would try to change his approach.

To ensure that the implied terms of the contract of employment are fulfilled on both sides, there are certain forms of conduct required, as set out in Box 2.2.

Box 2.2: Examples of implied terms – employers

- do not treat employees in an arbitrary or vindictive manner (see Example 2.3)
- offer to meet any legitimate expenses incurred by the employee on behalf of the employer, for example travelling expenses while representing the practice at an outside meeting
- provide details of an employee's service to a new employer. Although there is no law that requires references to be provided, employers are expected to confirm the basic details of an ex-employee's employment
- provide support to employees, for example ensuring staff have the appropriate training, equipment and level of workload to do their jobs
- inform employees of important decisions (see Example 2.2)
- refrain from issuing orders to employees to commit unlawful acts, such as falsifying accounts or medical records
- do not vary the contract unilaterally, i.e. without consultation, to the detriment of the employee. For example, announcing a reduction in holiday leave entitlement without consulting and gaining agreement with staff
- do not undermine an employee
- provide a non-smoking work environment

Examples of the implied terms for employees are set out in
Box 2.3.

Box 2.3: Rules for fulfilling implied terms – employees

- co-operate with the employer
- be ready and willing to work
- take care of the employer's property
- do not disclose any confidential information from the organisation
- obey reasonable and lawful instructions
- exercise reasonable care and skill
- act in good faith and fidelity
- co-operate and adapt to reasonable changes
- maintain a relationship of loyalty, mutual trust and fidelity

Custom and practice

Terms may be implied in employment contracts if they are
regularly adopted in a particular trade or industry or in a particular locality. For instance, a practice which regularly, over a
number of years, gives Christmas bonuses cannot withdraw this
benefit without first gaining consent from staff to what is in
effect a change to their contracts. Although such bonuses may
not be written into the contract, the custom and practice of
providing bonuses firmly establishes it as part of the contract
(*Frisehars Ltd v Taylor*, 1979 EAT 386/79). This point is further
exemplified in Example 2.4, which illustrates how custom and
practice can override the written terms of the contract in certain
circumstances.

Example 2.4

A practice had a retirement age of 60 years and this was written into
everyone's statement of terms and conditions of employment. However,
when staff approached the retirement age the practice often disregarded
it and allowed staff to work beyond 60. This flexibility caused no problem

until one of the receptionists aged 59, with whom the practice had experienced a lot of difficulties in the past, was given 3 months' notice of her impending retirement. She protested and asked to be allowed to continue working as others had before her. The practice refused, insisted that she leave on her 60th birthday and was then taken to an employment tribunal by the receptionist for unfair dismissal.

The practice lost the case because they could not demonstrate that 60 years was the normal retirement age. Their laxity over the years in adhering to the set age had undermined the written term in the contract of employment.

Customs and practices are often quite quickly established in organisations and it is wise to be aware that where a particular practice is introduced it may, once consistently established, become part of the contract of employment.

Incorporated terms

These refer to the express incorporation of terms determined by national and/or local collective agreements struck with recognised trades unions representing the employees.

Statutory terms

These are the legal provisions relating to employment relationships. The contract of employment will only override these if it exceeds the statutory minimum employment rights of the employee. For example, pregnant employees with less than one year's service are legally entitled to receive 18 weeks' maternity leave. A practice may be more generous and decide to specify 30 weeks' maternity leave for such staff. What it cannot do is specify less than 18 weeks. As legislation covering such statutory terms is introduced, so the contract of employment changes automatically.

Summary

A contract of employment therefore involves more than the written terms. Although reducing the main terms and conditions to writing is essential, it is necessary to recognise its limitations. No written statement, however detailed, can hope to be entirely comprehensive. There will always be certain areas of your relationship with your staff that cannot be codified but that nevertheless form an integral part of the total contract. There are many understandings between you and your staff that reflect goodwill and 'give and take', which cannot and should not be documented.

However, it is very important that as many as possible of the key elements of the terms and conditions are written and agreed. Introducing changes at a later date is far more difficult (and can be expensive) than putting them into the contract before the employee commences work.

There is one crucial aspect of contracts that must not be forgotten. When a new employee starts work, organisations must recognise — because employment tribunals and judges certainly do — that employers have more power at this point in the employment relationship than the employee. Terms agreed at this time, which are clearly unfair and to the disadvantage or detriment of the employee, may be deemed invalid and non-enforceable if later challenged through a tribunal.

Knowledge of the contract of employment is important in achieving an understanding of the complex and subtle area of illegal discrimination in employment. An employer's actions or omissions, and how these can breach both the contract of employment and discrimination law, is the key factor which employment tribunals address when faced with a claim of discrimination. Chapters 3 and 4 look at this whole area of discrimination, equal opportunities and the actions general practices can take to avoid litigation and promote equal opportunities in the workplace.

3
Discrimination

All stages of what we described in the introduction as the 'employment journey' can have a discriminatory element, either potential or real. Chapter 1 has already demonstrated that avoiding illegal discrimination is one of the most sensitive and daunting aspects of the management of people. It is appropriate therefore that it is the subject of these early chapters.

Since the 1960s, industrial relations in the UK have changed from a situation where employment law could be ignored, where legal actions were few and far between, into a more litigious society where the number of legal claims is increasing and in which the law is far more complex. However, good management of people demands far more than mere compliance with legal requirements. The real skill of management in this area is not merely to avoid breaking the law but to recognise the intrinsic organisational benefits of developing a non-discriminatory workplace.

Simply put and quoting from the equal opportunities pack from the Department of Education and Employment (1999a):

The UK ... is a multiracial society. It is also a society in which women account for nearly half of the working population. And increasingly it is being recognised that people with disabilities can make a full contribution to working life. Yet people from these groups frequently suffer unfair discrimination in employment .... Equal opportunities is a natural and integral part of good management practice, aimed at developing people to the fullest extent possible for the good of their organisations and of themselves.

Actively ensuring that people do not suffer discrimination also produces business advantages and is a far more effective approach than viewing non-discrimination as a rather vague social duty. The changes in the demography and gender composition of the UK workforce has led many employers to look at ways of positively attracting and retaining certain sectors of the community. The introduction of family-friendly policies, paternity leave, generous maternity leave and pay, abolishing age barriers and encouraging disabled people in recruitment and promotion all help the modern primary healthcare organisation compete for and retain skilled staff.

Clearly, before an employer embarks on such a review of and improvements to discriminatory or potentially discriminatory practices and policies, it is crucial to attain a basic understanding of the legal rules and principles which affect the employment relationship.

This chapter addresses these principles and Chapter 4 goes on to look at ways of creating a non-discriminatory workplace environment, including the thorny area of harassment and bullying at work.

The main principles of the laws covering discrimination

Discrimination at work involves treating some people less favourably than others on the basis of characteristics that are irrelevant to their ability to do the job in question. Such discrimination may be based on prejudiced stereotypes, for example viewing women with young children as unreliable, black people as lazy, disabled people as not fitting in with the organisation.

Discriminatory practices may also arise because an employer fails to take account of real differences between individuals, for example women do become pregnant and disabled people may need extra facilities. With the exception of ex-offenders, there is no qualifying period of employment before an individual can exercise his or her legal right not to be discriminated against.

This chapter focuses on those aspects of discrimination most relevant to primary healthcare, namely sex, race and disability discrimination. However, it also includes reference to discrimination on grounds of trade union membership, criminal record and age.

Sex and race discrimination

The law

As the main principles of both the sex and race discrimination acts are very similar they are taken together in this first section. The two main pieces of legislation relating to race and sex discrimination are the Sex Discrimination Act 1975 (SDA) and the Race Relations Act 1976 (RRA).

The law on racial discrimination was modelled on and closely followed the SDA. The case law on sex discrimination is good authority for interpreting the parallel provisions on race discrimination and vice versa. The Commission for Racial Equality (CRE) has similar powers and functions to the Equal Opportunities Commission (EOC) and both bodies have issued Codes of Practice for employers, providing guidance in avoiding unlawful practices and promoting equal opportunities in the workplace (CRE 1983; EOC 1985).

The SDA and RRA outlaw discrimination at all stages of the employment process from recruitment to dismissal. Between these two points, other stages involve terms and conditions of employment, access to promotion, transfer or training or any other benefits, facilities or services. Unlike other employment protection legislation, the Acts cover people other than straightforward job applicants and employees. They include the self-employed and independent contractors. As long as there is a contractual relationship, the Acts apply, for example to the process of appointing partners to a general practice.

The Codes of Practice are crucial to ensuring that employers avoid such discrimination and are admissible as evidence in any legal proceedings and must be taken into account by tribunals.

If a person feels they have been discriminated against then redress can be sought through an employment tribunal. Tribunals can order employers to amend their practices, to seek advice from the EOC/CRE and award compensation. There is no limit to the amount of compensation and some awards have been in excess of £100 000 and take into account injury to feelings.

Many organisations are unaware that for tribunals, in arriving at a judgement, the employer's motive is irrelevant. If the treatment is found to be based on sex or racial grounds, even if there was no intention to discriminate, the employer will lose the case.

What is sex and race discrimination?

Both Acts cover direct and indirect discrimination. Section 2(1) of the SDA is written as applying to women and is to be read as applying equally to the treatment of men.

Direct sex discrimination is where a person treats a woman less favourably than he or she would a man on grounds of her sex, or a married person less favourably than an unmarried person of the same sex on the grounds of marital status. The Act also applies to a man who is treated less favourably than a woman. It is also worth mentioning here that discriminating against a woman on the grounds of her pregnancy or any other maternity-related reason, is direct discrimination. This includes failing to appoint the best candidate (or withdrawing a job offer) on the grounds that the candidate is pregnant.

Direct race discrimination is where a person treats someone on racial grounds less favourably than they treat or would treat another person. The term race includes colour, race, nationality, ethnic or national origins. Discrimination on grounds of religion is unlawful in Northern Ireland.

Indirect discrimination is where an unjustifiable requirement or condition is applied equally to both sexes, but has a disproportionately adverse effect on one sex because the proportion of one sex that can comply with it is considerably smaller than the proportion of the other sex. The indirect race discrimination clauses under the RRA are broadly similar to those in the SDA. Examples of indirect discrimination can include:

- applying an unjustifiable age barrier; Chapter 1 contains an example of inappropriate wording of an advertisement and illustrates how this can constitute indirect sex discrimination
- promoting according solely on length of service (commonly known as 'buggins turn') rather than considering the merits of all potential candidates
- rigidly insisting on certain educational qualifications or abilities not essential to performance of the job. An example would be requiring a good command of spoken English for a warehouse porter who has no contact with the public
- selecting advertising media and/or publications to which sectors of society covered by the above Acts would not normally have access. A common discriminatory medium is advertising at the factory gate to which only current employees or their family and friends have access.

Discrimination in recruitment

Advertising

The main pitfall to be avoided in this area is in informal recruitment methods, where jobs are offered to individuals without being widely advertised or through word of mouth. These can have a discriminatory impact, tending to reproduce the existing sex and race balance of the workforce, reinforcing stereotypes and assumptions about the sort of person who can do the job.

Apart from certain circumstances (see the next section below), it is unlawful to engage in 'positive discrimination', which is appointing or promoting people solely because they are from an ethnic minority or they are of a sex which is under-represented in the workplace. However, it is lawful to encourage certain applicants to apply for a job, for example women or members of an ethnic minority, if there were no, or comparatively few, people of that racial group or sex doing the work in question in the UK, or within a given area, within the last 12 months. Such applicants can be encouraged, explicitly, to apply for a vacancy. However, to select for interview or be offered a job on the basis of their sex or race would constitute 'positive discrimination' and therefore would be unlawful.

Genuine occupational qualification

There is one area where positive discrimination is lawful and that is where there is a genuine need to recruit persons of one sex or a particular race. Such need is called a genuine occupational qualification (GOQ). The courts interpret such a qualification narrowly as it is a derogation from the principle of equal treatment.

Race

Discrimination in recruitment or promotion is permissible in cases where being of a particular racial or ethnic group or nationality is a GOQ. Section 5(2) of the RRA 1976 sets out the three grounds on which race can amount to a GOQ:

- participation in a dramatic performance or other entertainment, as a model in the production of a work of art or visual image where a person of the particular racial group is required for reasons of authenticity. For example, putting on a play about the apartheid era in the South Africa would require the employment of black actors
- the job involves serving food and drink in a particular setting and a member of a racial group is required for reasons of authenticity, e.g. the staffing of an Indian restaurant
- the job involves providing persons of a particular racial group with personal services promoting their welfare, and those services can be provided most effectively by a person of that racial group.

Sex

Section 7 of the SDA states that a job may be restricted to one sex where the essential nature of the job, or of particular duties attached to the job, calls for a member of one sex. This GOQ can only be claimed in relation to certain circumstances relating to the job, including privacy and decency (Section 7(2)(b)).

A GOQ maybe claimed where it is necessary to preserve privacy and decency if:

- the job is likely to involve physical contact (this means actual touching) with a person of the opposite sex who might reasonably object to the job-holder being of the other sex
- the job-holder is likely to work in circumstances where persons of the other sex are in a state of undress or using sanitary facilities and they might reasonably object to the job-holder being of the opposite sex.

An example would be where a practice has identified a real need to provide a female doctor for female patients and, crucially, there is no female partner. A GOQ could not be used to advertise for a female partner if the practice had a female doctor to whom the practice's female patients had access.

When considering whether a vacancy comes under the GOQ provision, employers should contact the EOC or CRE as appropriate, who will provide detailed advice on how to proceed with the advertising and recruitment. Such advice will include quoting in the advertisement the relevant section of the Act and that a GOQ applies to the post. If the advertisement is challenged in law, the burden of proof lies with the employer to establish the validity of a GOQ by providing substantiating evidence.

Training

Training is a key element of equal opportunities. The Acts make it unlawful to discriminate in access to training and that includes any form of education or instruction. Training, however, is the other area where the SDA permits positive discrimination, i.e. treating women differently and more favourably than men. Under Section 48 of the SDA, an employer is permitted to provide women only with access to training facilities to fit them for a particular kind of work as long as there were no women, or relatively few, doing the work in question within the previous 12 months. This is about encouraging women, and no guarantee of a job can be given as discrimination at the point of selection is always unlawful.

A common example of this positive action in the area of training can be found in the education sector. Far fewer women primary teachers, proportionately, apply for headships in comparison to male primary teachers. In recognition of this imbalance, some local education authorities offer 'women only' training courses to encourage and help their female teachers to apply for these posts when they are advertised.

Dismissal

Dismissing an employee on the grounds of sex or race is a clear case of unlawful discrimination. The most common form of discrimination in dismissing a person is indirect discrimination; for instance an employer who uses part-time work as a selection criterion for redundancy where three-quarters of the workforce are women working part time is discriminating unlawfully. Similarly, it would also be unlawful to use absence records which include maternity absence as a selection criterion for redundancy.

Retirement

It is permissible to have different retirement ages between different categories of workers but not between the sexes, although indirect discrimination can occur if one category with a higher age is predominantly one sex. For example, having different retirement ages based on status, and where the managers of the organisation are predominantly male and the rest of the workforce is predominantly female, could be discriminatory.

Equal pay

The Equal Pay Act was introduced in 1975 to help close the gap between men and women's earnings. The Act, and as later amended by the European Court of Justice, provides for women to claim equal pay where the work is the same or rated as equivalent or of equal value to that done by men.

Disability discrimination

What is disability?

The Disability Discrimination Act 1995 (DDA) defines disability as a physical or mental impairment (mobility, manual dexterity, physical co-ordination, speech, hearing or eyesight) which has a substantial and long-term adverse effect on the person's ability to carry out normal day-to-day activities. Mental impairment includes only those disabilities resulting from clinically well-recognised illnesses such as depression, while 'long-term effects' are those which have lasted at least 12 months or can reasonably be expected to last at least that long.

Severe disfigurement is seen as having a substantial adverse effect and therefore comes within the scope of the Act as does an impairment that is controlled or corrected by, for example, medication, artificial limbs or hearing aids. However, sight impairment that can be corrected by spectacles or contact lenses is outside the scope of the Act.

Progressive conditions, such as HIV infection, cancer and multiple sclerosis, are to be regarded as disabilities before they have had a substantial effect on normal day-to-day activities, as long as the condition is ultimately expected to result in such an effect.

This Act gives people with disabilities the right not to be discriminated against in employment, as well as a right to access to goods and services.

However, under this Act employment protection is only given to those who work for an employer who employs 15 or more staff.

The terms of the DDA

The Act makes it unlawful to discriminate against current or prospective employees with disabilities because of a reason relating to their disability unless the discrimination can be justified (see p. 48). Protection is given not only to job applicants and employees but also to apprentices and people who contract personally to provide services. The law covers people who are currently disabled as well as those who have had a disability in the past.

People who wish to seek compensation for unlawful discrimination can seek remedies through employment tribunals and these remedies are the same as under other discrimination legislation. ACAS is able to intervene as it would in other employment complaints.

What does it cover?

As with the SDA and RRA, under the DDA, employers must not discriminate in the recruitment and selection process, terms and conditions of employment, in the opportunities for promotion, transfer, training or other benefits, or in dismissal procedures.

The Act also requires employers to make 'reasonable adjustment' to working arrangements or the workplace where that would have overcome the practical effects of a disability. In interpreting 'reasonable adjustment', tribunals expect employers to be imaginative; adjustments include changes to the workplace or to the way in which the work is done. Box 3.1 gives examples.

Box 3.1: Reasonable adjustments

- making adjustments to premises
- allocating some duties to others
- transferring the person to fill an existing vacancy
- altering hours of work
- allowing the person to be absent for rehabilitation, assessment or treatment
- training
- acquiring or modifying equipment
- providing a reader or interpreter
- providing supervision

It must be remembered that in determining what is a 'reasonable adjustment' the size of the organisation and the resources available to it are taken into account. Examples 3.1 and 3.2, taken from tribunal cases, illustrate this point.

Example 3.1

The applicant had cerebral palsy and required assistance when dressing, eating and using the toilet. He was offered a job by Hampshire Constabulary, subject to it being able to make appropriate arrangements for his care needs. Despite intensive efforts, it proved impossible for the Hampshire Constabulary to make such arrangements, particularly in relation to using the toilet. The job offer was withdrawn and the Employment Appeal Tribunal ruled that the employer had not acted unlawfully.

Kenny v Hampshire Constabulary (1998) The Times, 22 October. Employment Appeal Tribunal.

Example 3.2

Mrs E Abbot was a primary school teacher and registered as blind. When her classroom assistant, Mrs Thomas, left, she was not replaced and Mrs Abbot found it very difficult to do her job. She resigned in June 1997 on health grounds of depression and stress. She took her case to a tribunal on the grounds that she had been discriminated against because of her disability. The tribunal agreed and awarded her £60 000 in damages.

Abbott v Waltham Forest Local Education Authority (2000) *Guardian,* 5 July. Employment Tribunal.

Unlike the SDA and RRA where there is no justification for discrimination, the DDA allows employers to discriminate against disabled people if such treatment is relevant to the circumstances of the individual case and the reason for the treatment is a substantial one. Example 3.1 above illustrates this point. A minor or trivial reason would not count as substantial. Employers do not have to make changes if the disabled person only experiences a minor disadvantage, they do not know that a person has a disability (and it is reasonable that they do not know) and the change required to overcome the disadvantage is not reasonable.

Age discrimination

There is no law against age discrimination in employment in the UK. However, in June 1999 the government published a voluntary code of practice *Age Diversity in Employment* (Department of Education and Employment 1999b) together with implementation guidance. The government has warned that if employers continue to discriminate on grounds of age, and specifying an age or age group in an advertisement is clear evidence of such discrimination, then the Code will be replaced by legislation. Chapter 1 gives further details of this Code and an example of a discriminatory advert (see page 15).

In fact, it is probably more effective to adopt an equal opportunities approach. It is much safer to focus, in both the advertisement and the selection process, on applicants' objective qualities, such as level and length of relevant professional experience, rather than such a blunt and unreliable indicator of job suitability as age.

Trade union membership

Until the Employment Relations Act 1999 (ERA), there was no right to trade union recognition. However, with the ERA and following certain conditions, employers with 21 or more staff must recognise trade unions for the purposes of negotiating on pay, hours and holidays. Any other terms and conditions can be included only at the agreement of both parties. Chapter 5 gives further details of this new recognition law.

The right not to be discriminated against on the grounds of membership or non-membership of a trade union was introduced in the early 1990s. Such victimisation would have been unheard of in primary care because trade unions have hardly figured in industrial relations in this sector. As there is likely to be a rise in the number of staff in primary healthcare who will become members of a trade union, the right not to be discriminated against on these grounds will take on a new significance.

Ex-offenders

Many employers are unwilling to take on someone with a criminal record, exhibiting a blanket prejudice regardless of the type of crime involved, the punishment delivered and how long ago it happened. Protection against such discrimination for ex-offenders is contained in the Rehabilitation of Offenders Act 1974.

The purpose of the Act is to allow some ex-offenders to put their criminal record behind them after a certain period of rehabilitation. The conviction is then 'spent'. The details of the rehabilitation periods are contained in Section 5 of the Act and are summarised in Box 3.2. Broadly, any prison sentence of two years six months or more cannot become 'spent' under the terms of the Act.

Box 3.2: Summary of rehabilitation periods under the Rehabilitation of Offenders Act 1974

Sentence	Rehabilitation period [†]
Absolute discharge	Six months
Probation, conditional discharge, bind over, care or supervision order	One year from conviction or on the date the order expires – whichever is the later
Fine or community service	Three years*
Imprisonment/youth custody of less than six months	Seven years*
Imprisonment/youth custody of six to 30 months	10 years*

[†] The rehabilitation period runs from the date of conviction.
*The rehabilitation period in these cases is halved for those persons who were under 17 years of age at the date of the conviction.

Once a conviction has become 'spent' then the individual must be treated as if there has been no criminal record. This means that the person can answer questions about criminal convictions and exclude any 'spent' convictions in their reply. If an employer subsequently learns of a spent conviction, there is no redress against the employee as it was a legitimate withholding of information.

The Act does not specify any remedies for the aggrieved job applicant or dismissed employee. The only recourse if they suffered dismissal in these circumstances, would be to invoke unfair dismissal proceedings (see Chapter 9). However, unlike other forms of unlawful discrimination, the employee would need one year's service before lodging such a claim at a tribunal.

Of most interest to primary care are the exempt occupations where the provisions of the Act do not apply. These are contained in the Rehabilitation of Offenders Act 1974 (Exceptions) Order. Broadly, these involve occupations where a high degree of trust, confidence, probity and integrity is demanded in the occupation and mainly relate to the medical and legal professions. They include doctors, dentists, nurses, midwives, opticians, pharmacists, social workers, teachers, youth workers, the police, prison service employees, traffic wardens, lawyers and judges. In these occupations, therefore, applicants and employees should answer any questions in relation to past convictions truthfully and the employer can take previous convictions into account without running foul of the law.

Preventing discrimination

The legal principles detailed above may look daunting. However, employers do not have to remember every detail in order to remain within the law, although it is important to be aware that legal cases are time-consuming and expensive, both emotionally and financially. There are no maximum limits on awards for cases of discrimination and the costs of defending legal proceedings can be considerable.

Therefore, the most important actions in creating a non-discriminatory work environment are the development, introduction, implementation and monitoring of an equal opportunities policy with, crucially, employment procedures which support and reflect the spirit of the policy. Tribunals are paying increasing attention to the employer's equal opportunities policy and comparing what actually happened with the procedures laid down in the employer's policy. Failure to follow one's own policy can be cited as evidence of a lack of commitment to equal opportunities and can strengthen the employee's claim against the employer.

A draft equal opportunities policy, written for a general practice, can be found in Appendix A. A policy on the associated area of preventing harassment in the workplace can be found in Appendix B and, as this is such a tricky area, it is the subject of the next chapter. However, before moving on to that area, there follow some examples of employment procedures which need to be in place if an equal opportunities policy is to be meaningful.

Recruitment and selection

Chapter 1 describes how to devise a selection procedure which would be as objective as possible and free from illegal discrimination. Here are some other points to note.

Preparatory paperwork

It is important to avoid the use of sexist job titles and to scrutinise personal specifications. Also these documents should avoid factors such as attitude and personality. Rather they should be drawn up to be as specific as possible and relevant to the requirements of the job. As shown in Chapter 1, emphasising such requirements as 'recent experience' may exclude women applicants who have been out of the workforce raising a family.

It is important to take care not to require higher levels of educational attainment than are necessary for the job in question, as this may exclude candidates who have been educated in another country. Similarly, if a practice only considers candidates with UK qualifications, this too may have an indirectly discriminatory effect.

Application forms should not ask applicants for information irrelevant to the job. It does not matter if a person is married or has children. Including such questions can be hard to justify as directly relevant to the job, if challenged at tribunal.

Interviews

Chapter 1 deals in detail with the methods and processes that ensure objectivity in the selection of candidates. To emphasise this, Box 3.3 includes the EOC advice to organisations on this subject.

Box 3.3: EOC advice on ensuring objectivity in the selection of candidates

1 All those involved in interviewing should be trained in the avoidance of illegal discrimination.

2 Interviews should be conducted by a panel and not by one interviewer.

3 Although it is not unlawful to ask questions about marital status or childcare arrangements, such questions may be taken as evidence of a discriminatory attitude. Such questions should never be asked unless they are strictly relevant to the job. For example, in the case of *Riches v Express Dairy Ltd* (1992) IRLR 564, a part-time woman employee applied for a full-time supervisor's post. At the interview she was questioned about her childcare arrangements and asked how she proposed to manage when her children were ill. She did not get the promotion and the tribunal held that these were questions that arose 'from the assumption which is still prevalent in many circles, that women are less reliable [than men] when it comes to time keeping'.

4 It is important that notes are taken at every stage of the selection process. A comprehensive record with reasons for decisions made should be kept of each interview conducted. It is essential if the organisation is later challenged by a tribunal. Tribunals are frequently inferring discriminatory conduct from an employer's failure to keep such records.

Discrimination during employment

Promotion opportunities

A claim of discrimination is far less likely if promotion opportunities are advertised as open to all suitably qualified applicants, with a formal recruitment and selection procedure as suggested in Chapter 1. Relying on an informal process can reinforce existing sex and race ratios and can exclude certain sectors from more senior jobs.

This point is illustrated by the case of *Schofield v Double Two Ltd.* (1992) Case No. 54582/91. Ms Schofield was a trainee supervisor. Her male colleague, also a trainee, was offered the post of assistant manager. The post was never advertised and therefore Ms Schofield had no opportunity to apply for it. The employer lost the case. One of the reasons it was lost was because the employer had not paid any regard to the Code of Practice on the elimination of sex discrimination (EOC 1985), particularly paragraph 25(d), which states that 'when general ability and personal qualities are the main requirements for promotion to a post, care should be taken to consider favourably candidates of both sexes with differing career patterns and general experience'.

4
Harassment and bullying at work

This chapter looks at the sensitive issue of harassment and bullying in the workplace and its place in the context of equal opportunities. It also addresses the fundamental need for all organisations, no matter how unpalatable it may first appear, to plan and anticipate claims of bullying and harassment and thereby put in place the tools which will not only help prevent such incidents but also guide the employer if such allegations occur.

Harassment is not only confined to sexual harassment, but can involve other forms of discrimination. Because it normally involves inter-personal relationships between two or more people, it can be fraught with emotion and prejudice, and gives rise to subjectivity and cloudy thinking.

The reason this aspect of discrimination is given such importance is because encouraging people to work to their maximum potential is one of the fundamental responsibilities of any manager. This responsibility is made extremely difficult, if not impossible, if there is bullying or harassment in the workplace. A general practice can, through the nature of the work, be a very stressful place to work. If there is also internal bullying or harassment then it can be a very unpleasant environment for both management and staff.

To underline this, a recent Nuffield Trust (Walsh 1998) report estimated that sick leave costs the NHS £700 million a year. As one of the most common responses to being harassed or bullied is to take time off work through sickness, these absence statistics are pertinent. The significance of the problem has been revealed by the first comprehensive survey of workplace bullying (Cooper and Hoel 2000). The survey found that one in four employees stated that they had been bullied in the past five years. This survey of 5300 workers, the largest of its kind ever carried out, defined bullying as:

> long-term and persistent negative behaviour ranging from abuse, humiliation and ridicule to the imposition of unmanageable workloads, unreasonable deadlines and continual fault finding.

The authors found that victims ranged from senior managers to shop floor workers, but that 75% of bullies were managers. Bullying was worse in the public sector than in the private sector. Funded by the British Occupational Health Research Foundation, the survey further found that victims took an extra seven days off work per year compared with other workers.

What is harassment?

A clear understanding of what constitutes harassment — how it happens, who does it, who experiences it and its effects — is a pre-requisite to developing any policies or procedures in this area.

Harassment will normally be a pattern of behaviour which continues over a period of time and which is unwanted, unreciprocated and uninvited by the recipient. Harassment affects the dignity of men and women at work. People can be subject to undignified behaviour on a wide variety of grounds including:

- gender, sexual orientation, AIDS/HIV, health (including disabilities, sensory impairments or learning difficulties)
- race, ethnic origin, nationality, skin colour and accent
- willingness to challenge harassment or bullying leading to victimisation

- membership or non-membership of a trade union
- age, physical characteristics, personal beliefs.

Harassment can be bullying and intimidatory behaviour that often stems from unknown factors, as well as those listed above. Examples of behaviour that may constitute harassment are set out in Box 4.1.

Box 4.1: Examples of harassment

- *physical harassment* – unwanted touching or petting, pinching or unnecessarily brushing against someone, physical assault and enforced sexual attention
- *verbal harassment* – persistent name-calling, sexual propositioning, making offensive comments or jokes, gossip, slander, sectarian songs and letters
- *non-verbal harassment* – displaying offensive posters or material and writing graffiti. Displaying emblems, symbols and flags, which may be offensive to particular religious or other ethnic/national groups
- *electronic harassment* – doing any of the above through computerised equipment, the most common being sending messages to another through e-mail
- *other anti-social behaviour* – isolation or non-co-operation, exclusion from social activities, ignoring the person, staring. Coercion for sexual favours and pressure to participate in political/religious groups. Intrusion by pestering, spying and stalking

It is very important to remember that it is not the intention of the perpetrator that defines whether harassment has occurred but whether the behaviour is unacceptable by normal standards and disadvantageous to the complainant. In this respect, it is essential to distinguish between a manager's legitimate right to discuss concerns (or even discipline a person) about their performance or conduct from bullying or harassment. Similarly, it is important to distinguish between sexual relationships freely entered into, and acceptable to those involved, and sexual harassment.

Sexual harassment

The sensitivity of the most common and most complex form of harassment, sexual harassment, justifies a more detailed discussion here.

Dealing with and preventing sexual harassment does not mean that mutually acceptable friendships or flirtation are outlawed. Rather, it is about the creation and maintenance of a work environment where everyone is treated professionally and with respect. It is about being a good employer and staying within the law.

The exact nature of sexual harassment can vary in each individual case. However, there are three general principles which help define sexual harassment.

The first principle is that sexual harassment is unwanted, unreciprocated conduct which is uninvited and not welcomed. It is behaviour that is imposed on another in some way.

The second principle, which follows from the first, is that it is for the recipient to determine what constitutes harassing behaviour. It is the effect of the behaviour and not the motives of the perpetrator that is the determining factor. Therefore behaviour which is acceptable in one context could be sexual harassment in another.

The third principle is that sexual harassment is related to gender or sexual orientation. It can often be (but does not have to be) conduct which is 'sexual' in terms of it being related to the sexual act and/or behaviour aimed at initiating sexual relations. It can also be behaviour that is offensive or intimidatory to an employee because of his/her gender or sexual orientation. A description of harassment is illustrated in Example 4.1.

Example 4.1

Linda Jones, the practice's manager, called a meeting of the partners to inform them that Katy Rowan, a receptionist, had complained that Doug

Harvey, a physiotherapist, had been over-familiar. Katy alleged that Doug made personal remarks about her appearance, insisted on calling her darling and had started to enquire about her boyfriend.

The partners were very concerned. One of them wondered what the practice could do as Doug was employed by the local Trust and not the practice. Linda informed them that Katy had not asked Doug to stop his behaviour as she was too embarrassed to say anything to him. But Katy had told Linda that she would resign if the behaviour didn't stop. Linda advised the partners that she could see a claim for constructive dismissal looming unless the matter was resolved, and quickly. After discussing the way they were going to handle the issue, they decided to make a formal complaint to the Trust and advise Katy of the fact. There was a realisation that the potential for litigation was considerable and the view, voiced by Linda, that what they should have done a long time ago was to develop a policy on harassment.

Harassment and bullying at law

It is now clear that the existence of an unpleasant and intimidating working environment is sufficient detriment to establish a case of harassment and, through the development of case law, harassment at work is unlawful under several Acts.

Sexual harassment can result in claims under the Sex Discrimination Act 1975 and the Employment Rights Act 1996, which covers unfair dismissal and constructive dismissal. Although there is no direct reference to sexual harassment in these Acts (and this applies to racial harassment under the Race Relations Act 1976), employees who suffer harassment may claim direct discrimination where it can be shown that the harassment 'constitutes a detriment', that is to say, the harassment demonstrably tells against the victim in a tangible way. Many employees successfully sue their employers in a tribunal where they are dismissed as a result of harassment, for example for refusing sexual advances. For a claim of sexual or racial harassment to succeed, the harassment (which includes abuse) must be related to the person's sex or race.

In addition, in Northern Ireland, religious harassment is protected by the Fair Employment (Northern Ireland) Acts 1976 and 1989. The Disability Discrimination Act 1995 protects people with disabilities against unfavourable treatment.

It is important to realise that employers are vicariously liable for the discriminatory actions of their employees even if the employer has no knowledge of, or has not sanctioned, such actions. Taking preventative measures — a clear policy against harassment for example — can be accepted as a defence against vicarious liability.

Employers can also be liable for the actions of third parties (people other than their own employees) where the third party has harassed an employee in circumstances which the employer could have controlled. The employer's direct and vicarious responsibility in this area is illustrated by the *Burton v De Vere Hotels* case (1996) IRLR 596. Waitresses were sexually and racially harassed by the entertainer Bernard Manning and some guests at a private hotel. The tribunal found that the employer had subjected his employees to harassment because he could have avoided or limited the harassment by following good employment practice. The hotel should have been alert from the start and acted from the first complaint, which may have included removing the waitresses or stopping the show. The implications for general practice are significant. Harassment of staff by others visiting the practice, for example pharmaceutical reps, the window cleaner or patients, can become the partnership's responsibility.

General harassment not specifically related to race or sex, such as bullying, is not currently protected by statute. However, employers may be liable if they behave in such a way themselves or if they fail to deal effectively with such behaviour because there are remedies at law. Examples of the way current legislation can be used by employees include the following.

- Under the Health and Safety at Work Act 1974, employers must take such steps as are reasonably practicable for the health and safety of all employees. If bullying in the workplace causes an employee physical harm or mental stress leading to illness, then the employer may be liable.

- An employee may resign because of a severe case of bullying or harassment and claim the employer is in fundamental breach of contract which entitles him or her to resign and regard himself or herself as having been dismissed. Shouting at staff in front of other employees or patients, persistent intimidatory behaviour or the regular use of sarcasm can all constitute sufficient grounds for an employee to resign and claim constructive (and therefore unfair) dismissal at a tribunal. Chapter 2 details the implicit terms of the contract of employment of trust and confidence and behaving reasonably, which, if breached by the employer, can lead to claims of constructive dismissal.

- Protection from Harassment Act 1997. This Act was designed to prevent stalking but it can also be used in serious cases of workplace harassment and both civil and criminal action can be taken.

- Under the Criminal Justice and Public Order Act 1994, behaviour or acts which intend the recipient to feel harassed, alarmed or distressed are illegal and can result in a custodial sentence of up to six months or a £5000 fine. This Act includes all kinds of harassment, including sex, race and disability. The Act covers the use of threatening, abusive or insulting words or behaviour, or disorderly behaviour and the display of any writing, sign or other visible representation that is threatening, abusive or insulting.

How to combat harassment

Changing the culture

First and foremost organisations need to develop a culture in which harassment and bullying are unacceptable, and if such behaviour occurs, individuals should have the confidence to bring complaints without fear of reprisals.

In Example 4.1, Linda had, of course, identified the most effective tool in dealing with this issue – the development of a policy. The very process of writing a policy and informing everyone of its contents can communicate what is deemed acceptable and unacceptable behaviour and provide the tool for preventing harassment and the procedure for dealing with allegations.

The best time to develop such a policy is before any incidents occur and not when an allegation has been made and the situation is 'hot'. A policy needs to have procedures for dealing with allegations both informally and formally. Very few people deliberately set out to harass others. Often an alleged harasser may be unaware that their behaviour is causing discomfort or offence and may stop if informed of its impact. The best person to deliver this message is the complainant at the time of the incident and so staff need to be encouraged to attempt to deal with the issue themselves. It keeps the problem from escalating. However, it must be recognised that confronting unacceptable behaviour in others is difficult. If the complainant cannot deal with it himself or herself, if the incident(s) are serious and/or if the alleged harasser is a person in a position of power (partner or practice manager, for example), then the policy needs to set out clearly, and in detail, how the issue is to be handled.

Developing and introducing a harassment policy

As has been made clear already, the key decision in preventing bullying and harassment is to design and introduce a policy on harassment. Such a policy sends a very clear message to everyone about what is and what is not acceptable behaviour; the training involved in introducing the policy reinforces the message.

The importance of this management tool cannot be underestimated. In addition to using it to promote equal opportunities and prevent harassment and bullying from occurring, there are other important reasons for having such a policy and its benefits are set out in depth in Box 4.2.

Box 4.2: Reasons for having a harassment policy

A harassment policy should address the following key areas:

- why the organisation is introducing the policy, including reference to the legal background, and a clear statement that the organisation will not tolerate harassment and bullying
- the scope of the policy – to whom it applies. In a general practice, this will be the partners and staff of the practice, with a codicil that although the policy cannot be applied to patients and other users of or suppliers to the practice, it maybe possible to counter harassment in other ways
- defining harassment with clear examples of what constitutes bullying and harassment
- the responsibilities of doctors and managers to implement the policy and ensure it is understood; the staff's responsibilities in its adherence
- the damaging effects on individuals and the practice of such behaviour and why it will not be tolerated
- the complaints procedure and its relation to the practice's disciplinary procedure
- a commitment to complainants that they will not be victimised for making a complaint
- monitoring processes to ensure that the harassment has stopped.

In summary the key reasons for a policy are that:

- trying to deal with a harassment allegation without a procedure is similar to dealing with an allegation of serious misconduct without a disciplinary procedure
- tribunals view the absence of a policy as inferring illegal discriminatory practices
- related to tribunal judgements is the principle of vicarious responsibility.

As stated earlier, anything done by a person in the course of his or her employment is treated by tribunals as having been done by the employer as well as by the employee, whether or not it was done with the employer's knowledge or approval. An employer has a good defence against such allegations of vicarious responsibility if the organisation took such steps as were reasonably practicable to prevent the employee from doing that act, or from doing, in the course of his or her employment, acts of that description. This defence is much easier to rely on if the employer has comprehensive equal opportunities policies, including procedures for dealing with harassment, as set out in Appendices A and B.

Tribunals now refer to the European Commission's Code of Practice for guidance on measures to combat sexual harassment. This Code has stated that as sexual harassment is linked to a woman's status at work, the most effective sexual harassment policy is likely to be one which is an integral part of a general equal opportunities policy, as described in Chapter 3.

The Code's recommendations for a policy include:

- a clear policy statement that harassment will not be permitted or condoned and that employees have the right to complain about it if it does occur
- the identification of what behaviour is not permitted
- placing a duty on management to implement the policy and ensure all managers and supervisors are trained in the policy
- explaining the procedure for complaining with reassurances about taking such complaints seriously
- communicating the policy effectively to all staff so that staff know who to complain to and perpetrators are aware of the consequences of their behaviour, which should include disciplinary action.

What to do if harassment is alleged

Initial steps

When writing a harassment policy the most difficult part can be designing the complaints procedure. As indicated earlier, harassment and bullying can involve personal issues and a lot of perpetrators are unaware that their behaviour is causing offence. Often a quiet word will stop the behaviour, and a complaints procedure needs to incorporate both informal and formal approaches. If there is no scope for both, then situations which could have been dealt with quickly, informally and kept low key, become formalised with all the trauma (and managerial time) that involves.

When harassment occurs, the first step is to ensure that the complainant has kept accurate and detailed notes of the incident(s). Information to be recorded by complainant should include:

- date of first and subsequent incidents of harassment
- location of incident
- nature of incident (to cover both actions and comments of the other party or parties)
- feelings of the person being harassed at the time(s) of the harassment
- names of any witnesses.

They also need to report the matter to someone in the practice who can deal with it; the practice manager would normally be the first person to deal with the allegation. However, a partner needs to be the investigator if it relates to the practice manager or another partner's behaviour.

As with a disciplinary issue (see Chapter 8), a full but discreet investigation needs to take place, after which the most appropriate action can be taken. Obviously the severity of the complaint, both in terms of incidents and frequency, will be the significant factor.

When a complaint is first made, it needs to be investigated swiftly and confidentially (if possible) while ensuring that the rights and dignity of all are preserved. Ignoring a complaint can lead to litigation, with the employer having little or no defence.

Depending on the result of the investigation, the action taken could range from getting an assurance from the harasser that there will be no repetition, to dismissal for gross misconduct (see Chapter 8).

Formal procedures

When it comes to a formal process, people need to know to whom they should make a formal complaint. Clearly in general practice this will be the practice manager or a designated partner. The investigation of the complaint will not be dissimilar to the process used for handling a disciplinary investigation (see Chapter 8).

The investigation should be prompt, thorough and impartial, with both parties being able to prepare and fully state their cases. As far as is possible and practicable the confidentiality of both parties and any witnesses should be preserved.

When a complaint is upheld, the procedure should include various options for resolving the issue. Such options can range from an apology from the perpetrator to invoking the practice's disciplinary procedure. The option selected will be determined by the severity and/or frequency or persistence of bullying or harassment and the views of the complainant. A common option is to transfer the perpetrator to some other part of the organisation. This option will be impractical for many practices, but if it is feasible then it needs to be included.

On this last point it is important to ensure that where the perpetrator is transferred, no breach of contract occurs, or a claim of constructive dismissal could arise. For example, transfers on disadvantageous terms and conditions of employment can be offered to the perpetrator but only where the allegations are proved and as an alternative to dismissal. If a complaint is not upheld, the consequences for staff relations can be significant and therefore in these circumstances the voluntary transfer of one of the employees should be considered.

Monitoring

It is important to check that the harassment has stopped. This can be done through various methods, including observing behaviour and interviewing the complainant.

Many organisations offer counselling support to both perpetrators and complainants. This counselling is often undertaken by counsellors external to the organisation. It may be tempting for one of the partners to undertake this counselling role. However, as harassment cases may later involve disciplinary action, it would be inappropriate, as a partner who earlier counselled an employee in confidence may then be involved in the decision to discipline that individual.

Reference in the policy should also be made to the action the practice will take against proven malicious and false allegations.

Training in the policy

It is insufficient to merely hand out the policy to staff. This area of employee relations is subtle and can be complex. It is important, therefore, to undertake a training seminar on the policy and its implications. The overt and covert benefits of the training include:

- the provision of information as to the policy's contents
- the ability of people to operate the policy
- greater understanding as to each person's personal and wider responsibility in preventing bullying and harassment and adhering to the policy
- reinforcement of the message to all about what is acceptable and what is not acceptable behaviour
- giving people the confidence to tackle harassment and bullying.

In conclusion, a harassment policy can help develop and reinforce a culture in which bullying and harassment are known to be unacceptable and where people are confident enough to confront it without fear of ridicule or victimisation. The introduction of and training in the policy helps to create a climate where harassment is unlikely and even if it does occur, the practice is equipped to deal with complaints promptly, effectively and fairly.

5
Employee rights

This chapter looks at individuals' employment rights, concentrating on those that are introduced under new legislation. For ease of reference, Appendix C summarises current rights and those introduced in 1999 and 2000.

In 1997, the new Labour administration undertook to shift some power away from the employer to the employee. These changes are contained in The Employment Relations Act 1999 (ERA). This Act represented a significant step in implementing the government's programme on individual employment rights and family-friendly policies. It has radically changed the way trade unions can obtain recognition and secure a place in even small organisations. The provisions of the Act have been brought into effect progressively; some provisions came into effect in autumn 1999 and others during the course of the following year.

The Act is divided into two distinct areas. First, the rights of the individual which we address first, as they are most likely to have an immediate impact on primary care and are of more interest to individual employees at the moment. The second area addresses the rights of trade unions to achieve recognition for the purposes of collective bargaining, in other words trade unions representing employees in negotiating with employers on the terms and conditions of employment in the workplace.

In addition to the ERA, there have been some other pieces of legislation affecting employees, most significantly law relating to whistle blowing, which are addressed under the section 'Other legislation'.

Individual rights

Unfair dismissal and compensation

The first change in legislation, and perhaps the one with the most immediate impact for practice staff, was the simple change in the qualifying period for claiming unfair dismissal. Until June 1999, employees had to have been employed by an employer for a minimum of two years before they were able to take action against the employer for unfair dismissal. This period is now reduced to one year (this change was reflected in the same reduction for qualifying for extended maternity leave; see pages 72–3).

This right to sue employers for unfair dismissal, after one year's service, also applies to claims of 'constructive dismissal'. This is where an employee feels that he or she has been forced to resign through the actions or omissions of the employer. Example 5.1 illustrates this.

Example 5.1

The senior partner of a three doctor practice introduced a staff appraisal scheme and insisted on conducting the appraisal interviews himself. The practice manager complained that this undermined her position with the staff. Also, as her career had previously involved appraisal interviewing, she was better qualified for the task. These complaints were ignored by the senior partner and he went ahead and arranged a time table of appraisal interviews with the staff.

The manager put her grievance in writing to the other two partners who duly investigated. In the grievance hearing they informed her that as the practice intended to introduce peer appraisal, it was important that one of the partners gain experience in this area. Despite the manager's threat that if she was excluded from the appraisal scheme she would resign, they endorsed the senior partner's decision to appraise the staff.

One week after the grievance hearing the practice manager resigned. However, before her notice period expired the partners sought advice and were informed that their behaviour had made the practice vulnerable to a claim of constructive dismissal. They hastily reviewed and over-turned their decision and the senior partner agreed to a more secondary role in the appraisal scheme. The practice manager withdrew her resignation although it took some time to regain her trust in and respect for the partners.

In addition to this change in the qualifying period, the maximum amount a tribunal can award in compensation has also changed.

The award of compensation is made to employees who have been proved to have been unfairly dismissed and is to compensate the employee for the actual losses they may have incurred as a result of such dismissal. While tribunals have a good deal of discretion, the compensatory award is not meant to be punitive and is calculated under certain heads of compensation. These are:

- immediate loss of earnings
- future loss of earnings
- expenses incurred as a result of the dismissal
- loss of employment protection and pension rights.

The maximum compensatory amount has been increased from £12 000 to £50 000 and from now on this amount will be index-linked. It is anticipated that this increase will have the effect of making tribunal action more attractive to higher-paid employees who do not find work for some time and who may have previously considered the £12 000 maximum too little to make it worth their while embarking on litigation.

Maternity rights

Given the preponderance of female employees in primary healthcare, the changes to maternity rights under the ERA are of particular relevance. Maternity legislation and the rules relating to notification of the pregnancy, taking maternity leave and returning to work are complex. Even though the aim of the ERA changes is to simplify the rules, they still remain complex. To further simplify them, we discuss the changes under the following headings:

- terminology
- summary of the changes
- notification of maternity leave
- compulsory maternity leave
- notification of return to work
- contacting employees on maternity leave
- sickness immediately following maternity leave
- returning to the same job.

Terminology

What was called 'basic maternity leave' is now called 'ordinary maternity leave'. What was called 'extended maternity leave' is now called 'additional maternity leave' and this amount has not changed. That is, a woman who qualifies for additional maternity leave can take up to a maximum of 11 weeks maternity leave before the expected week of confinement and up to 29 weeks after the birth, with an overall maximum period of maternity leave of 40 weeks.

Summary of the changes

The changes to the Act can be summarised as follows:

- the right for any pregnant employee, regardless of length of service, to take maternity leave has been in force for a number of years. This period of 'ordinary maternity leave' of 14 weeks is now increased to 18 weeks

- the qualifying service for women to take 'additional leave' has decreased from two to one year's service with the employer
- the employment rights and benefits retained by women on maternity leave have been clarified. Employees are able to continue to receive employee benefits, including seniority and pension rights but excluding remuneration
- changes have been made to notification periods and the right to return to the same job
- the rules relating to sickness following maternity leave have changed.

These changes to the Act apply to those employees whose expected week of childbirth began on or after 30 April 2000 and are now discussed in more detail.

Notification of maternity leave

Before taking maternity leave, the employee must give 21 days' notice (in writing, if requested by the employer) that she is pregnant, her expected week of childbirth and the date her leave is due to start. If requested, the employee must produce a certificate from a registered medical practitioner or midwife confirming the expected date of childbirth.

Compulsory maternity leave

This applies to women whose babies are born later than expected and where their maternity leave entitlement has expired before they have had time to recover from the birth. Employees are now prohibited from returning to work during the two weeks after the birth.

Notification of return to work

Previous to the ERA there were different rules depending on whether ordinary or additional maternity leave was taken, relating to the notice a woman had to give her employer before returning to work after taking maternity leave. These have now changed and the employee need only give notice if she intends to return to work *before* her maternity leave entitlement has been used. A minimum of 21 days' notice is required in such circumstances and the notice must specify the actual date she intends to return.

The employer may postpone the return where 21 days' notice has not been given and has no obligation to pay the employee if she does return earlier.

Contacting employees on maternity leave

Due to the length of maternity leave — a maximum of 40 weeks (see above) — a woman with one year's service can take, many employers wish to contact the employee to request confirmation of the date of childbirth and to find out if she still wishes to return to work. This wish to contact the employee is catered for in the legislation as follows:

- no request can be sent before 21 weeks of maternity leave have elapsed
- the employee must reply within 21 days (or as soon as practicably possible) if she wishes to retain her right to return to work
- in order to avoid any possible claims for unfair dismissal, the employer must ensure that the request for this information is accompanied by a statement setting out the employee's rights regarding the date of return, confirming the last possible date by which she must return and the consequences of failing to reply.

Sickness immediately following maternity leave

Previous to these changes in legislation, employees could extend their maternity leave on grounds of maternity-related illness. This no longer applies and normal sickness procedures apply following the date of return. This means that women who, due to illness, are not able to return to work on the due date automatically move from being on maternity leave to being on sickness leave and must be treated as any other employee taking sick leave.

Returning to the same job

Women are entitled to return from 'ordinary maternity leave' to the job they left when they took maternity leave. However, women returning from 'additional maternity leave' have the right to return to the same job or, if that is not reasonably practicable, to another suitable and appropriate job on terms and conditions which are no less favourable. Security of employment and pension rights are preserved for both categories of employees.

Parental leave

An important new right is that employees with one year's service with the employer and who are parents (including adoptive parents) have the right to 13 weeks' unpaid parental leave for the purpose of caring for the child. There is no obligation on the part of the employee to provide evidence that the parental leave is or was used to care for the child.

This right applies to all parents of children born or adopted after 15 December 1999. This right ceases once the child reaches the age of 5 years.

For part-time staff the right will be pro rata. For example, a member of staff who works two days a week will be entitled to 26 days leave; a week's leave means seven days' absence from work. The 13 weeks' leave applies to each individual child so that parents of twins, for example, are entitled to 26 weeks' parental leave.

The parental leave must be taken before the child's fifth birthday or within five years of adoption. Parents of disabled children can take the leave up until the child's 18th birthday – disability being determined by the receipt of the Disability Living Allowance.

If an employee is prevented by the employer from taking the leave or it is unreasonably delayed, the employee can complain to a tribunal within three months and compensation will be a combination of what is 'just and equitable' and compensation for any loss caused.

The regulations set out a model form of agreement, which is set out in Box 5.1 below. It describes the arrangements for taking parental leave and states that parental leave should be taken in a minimum of one-week blocks. For example, taking two days' parental leave will count as one week from the 13-week entitlement. The exception to this rule applies to the parents of disabled children. To meet the special needs of disabled children, their parents can take their parental leave in individual days.

This model form will apply in the absence of any collective or workforce agreement to the contrary. Therefore it is important for practices to agree (and it must be agreed and not enforced against the wishes of the staff) a form of parental leave that suits their own practice. Employers can be more generous than the regulations but not less generous, for example by imposing lower age limits or a later birth or adoption date.

Box 5.1: The model agreement as it would apply to a general practice

> If you wish to exercise your right to parental leave the following conditions apply:
>
> • evidence needs to be produced of your parental responsibility and the age of the child, e.g. birth certificate, court order, etc.

- you must give a minimum of 21 days' notice of when the parental leave is to begin and end.* Also, if the leave is for two weeks or less then at least four weeks' notice must be given and if for more than two weeks, the notice must be at least twice the number of weeks required, e.g. six weeks' notice for three weeks' leave
- parental leave cannot be taken in blocks of less than one week, therefore part of a week will count as one week
- employees can take no more than four weeks' leave in any one year
- if you are an expectant father or expecting to adopt a child, you must give at least 13 weeks' notice and specify the expected date of birth/ adoption of the child
- the practice has the right to postpone parental leave in certain circumstances, for up to six months. You will be given the reasons for the postponement and the appropriate notice of when you can take the leave. The notice period is the same as for employees (please see * above)
- you continue to be employed while on parental leave and the terms of your contract of employment of mutual trust and confidence continue while you are on parental leave. When you return to work you will be given the same job. If, for any reason, your parental leave has exceeded four weeks in any one year then you will be given the same job or, if this is not practicable, a suitable job on the same terms and conditions of employment

Although not included in the above model agreement, it would be wise to include in any practice agreement the rights, included in the Act, of parents of disabled children to take parental leave in individual days, if necessary, to meet the special needs of the child.

During the period of parental leave an employee's contract continues and obligations such as trust and confidence, good faith and confidentiality remain in place. Employees have the right to return to the same job or, if that is not reasonably practicable, to another suitable and appropriate job on terms and conditions that are no less favourable. Security of employment and pension rights are preserved.

There is no legal obligation for employers to keep records of parental leave. However, as an individual is only entitled to 13 weeks' leave per child, there is an obvious administrative responsibility on all employers to record parental leave and ensure that this record is sent to the employee's next employer. Similarly, it is necessary for employers to check the parental leave record of all new staff.

Right to time off for dependants

This regulation gives an employee the right to time off during working hours to deal with an emergency involving one of his or her dependants.

Under the regulations a dependant is defined as:

- a spouse
- a child
- a parent
- someone who cohabits with the employee but is not his or her employee, tenant, lodger or boarder
- someone who reasonably relies on the employee for assistance when ill, injured or for the provision of care.

In relatively small organisations such as general practices, most practice managers will have an accurate idea as to the people who are dependent – under the above definitions – on their staff.

Most good employers will give staff reasonable time off work to deal with or make arrangements to deal with a sudden family problem. This regulation gives legal legitimacy to good practice. It is based on the principle that employees are entitled to time off for dependants in order to:

- provide assistance when a dependant falls ill, gives birth, is injured or assaulted

- make provision for the care of an ill or injured dependant
- deal with the consequences of the death of a dependant
- deal with the situations where the care of a dependant has been unexpectedly disrupted or stopped, e.g. the nanny or childminder of an employee's child suddenly falls ill and there is no one to look after the child
- deal with an unexpected incident involving a child at school or other educational establishment.

The employee must tell his or her employer of the reason for the absence as soon as is reasonably practicable and give some idea as to how long he or she expects to be absent.

As with much employment legislation these regulations are peppered with the word 'reasonable'. There may be difficult issues to decide. For example, what is 'reasonable' time off and whether the time is to take 'necessary action'. Those practices that have a policy on time off to deal with such events will be able to use the policy to guide them through requests from staff. Those practices that have no policy with stated times should seriously consider developing one.

The regulations do not specifically state that the right to this time off is to be paid or unpaid. A refusal to pay may constitute a refusal to allow time off. Good management practice would dictate that given that the events which give rise to this time off are sudden, unanticipated and even traumatic, withholding salary for the time absent would be highly demotivating to both the individual concerned and other members of the team. Again a policy specifying how long such time off would be paid, unpaid, etc., will clarify these issues and ensure fairness to all staff, as well as help to ensure there is no abuse of the provisions. An example of specifying such time off might be:

a half-day's pay to make provision for the care of an ill or injured dependant and thereafter unpaid time off and at the discretion of the partnership/practice manager depending on the circumstances of the case.

Refusing to give time off may give rise to a complaint at an employment tribunal.

Disciplinary and grievance hearings

The changes within this area of an individual's rights have been incorporated into the ACAS Code on Disciplinary and Grievance Procedures, 2000 on employee representation. An employee now has the legal right to be accompanied by a trade union official, or some other representative from the workforce, at a serious disciplinary or grievance hearing. If the representative is not available to attend, the hearing can be postponed by up to a maximum of five working days.

A 'representative' is interpreted as a person who accompanies the employee but does not answer questions on the employee's behalf. Appendices D and E give examples of disciplinary and grievance procedures, respectively, which might be appropriate for general practice. Boxes 5.2 and 5.3 set out how a practice's disciplinary and grievance procedures could be amended to accommodate the new legal rights of employees.

Box 5.2: Disciplinary procedure

In any disciplinary interview or hearing which may result in a formal warning or other serious action, the employee has the right to be accompanied by a representative. If a member of a trade union, the employee may be accompanied by his or her trade union representative. If not a member of a trade union, the employee may be accompanied by a fellow employee of his or her choice.

The representative will be able to address the hearing and confer with the employee but they will not be able to answer questions on behalf of the employee.

The hearing will be postponed by up to a maximum of five working days if the employee's chosen representative is not available on the first occasion.

Box 5.3: Grievance procedure

Under stage/s ... where interviewing the employee forms part of the investigation, the employee will have the right to be accompanied by a representative. If a member of a trade union, the employee may be accompanied by his or her trade union representative. If not a member of a trade union, the employee may be accompanied by a fellow employee of his or her choice.

The representative will be able to address the hearing and confer with the employee but they will not be able to answer questions on behalf of the employee.

The hearing will be postponed by up to a maximum of five working days if the employee's chosen representative is not available on the first occasion.

Fixed-term contracts

The law relating to fixed-term contracts is complex and vulnerable to case law interpretation. It is helpful therefore to set out the law as it applied prior to the changes in the ERA in order to understand better the amendments introduced in 1999.

Fixed-term contracts are double-edged swords. They allow the employer to terminate employment at a future fixed date and, prior to 25 October 1999, as long as the appropriate 'waiver clause' was inserted into fixed term contracts for one year or longer, the employer was protected against a claim for unfair dismissal. This waiver provision has now been removed. This means that should a fixed-term contract for one year or more, entered into on or after 25 October 1999, not be renewed, the employer must treat the non-renewal as a dismissal and act accordingly (see Chapters 8 and 9) to avoid a claim for unfair dismissal.

It is still lawful to include a clause where the employee, on the non-renewal of a fixed-term contract of employment, waives his or her right to a redundancy payment. However, such redundancies should be treated with the same care as any other dismissal through reason of redundancy, if the employer is to avoid a claim for unfair dismissal.

Collective rights: trade union recognition

Although traditionally primary healthcare organisations have had little experience of organised labour, the NHS has a long history of collective bargaining and formalised industrial relations. Collective bargaining under the ERA is deemed to be the right of trade unions to represent employees in negotiating with employers on pay, hours and holidays. Any other terms and conditions can only be included at the agreement of both parties and after the trade union has gained recognition for collective bargaining.

Prior to the ERA, there was no legal obligation to recognise any trade union for any purpose; even if 100% of the workforce were members of a trade union, the employer could refuse to recognise the trade union. However, now the ERA enables trade unions to achieve recognition from organisations that employ 21 staff or more. Clearly many primary healthcare organisations fall into this category and individual practices will be approached by trade unions to this end.

What should a practice do if approached by a trade union to be recognised?

The trade union will make a formal written request for recognition. For a request to be legitimate, certain conditions apply. First, the union must have a certificate of independence, and second, the practice must employ at least 21 workers on the date the request is made or employ an average of at least 21 workers in the 13 weeks ending with the day the request was made.

Many practices will fall into this category and would have to take the request seriously. A period of 10 days is allowed, at the end of which the practice has three options:

- **Option 1 – recognise the trade union.** If 50% or more of the practice's staff are members of a trade union, the practice has little option but to recognise the trade union for collective bargaining purposes. However, this is not always straightforward, as the further options show. Both parties will agree a bargaining unit, i.e. the categories of staff for whom the trade union will represent and for whom they are entitled to conduct collective bargaining. A formal written agreement will then be negotiated and signed by both parties.
- **Option 2 – refuse the initial request but agree to negotiate further.** The parties may continue to conduct negotiations for a period of 20 days, which can be extended if both parties agree. The result of these negotiations will be either Option 1 or Option 3.
- **Option 3 – refuse recognition.** The employer may refuse to recognise the trade union either immediately the request is received or following the above 20-day negotiating period. If the trade union has a membership level of at least 10% of the proposed 'bargaining unit' it can refer the matter to the Central Arbitration Committee (CAC) which will become formally involved in the issue. There follows a period of 20 days (or longer if ordered by CAC) where CAC will attempt to help the employer and trade union to reach an agreement on the appropriate bargaining unit. If no such agreement is possible, the CAC will make a ruling on what is the appropriate bargaining unit within 10 days of the expiry of the 20-day period. In making such a ruling, the CAC is constrained by a list of criteria laid down in the Act. Box 5.4 sets out these criteria.

Box 5.4: Criteria for CAC decisions

- the need for the unit to be compatible with effective management
- the views of both parties
- existing national and local bargaining arrangements
- desirability of avoiding small, fragmented bargaining units within an organisation
- the characteristics of workers falling within the proposed bargaining unit and of any other employees whom the CAC considers relevant
- the location of the workers

Once the bargaining unit has been defined, it may be possible to resolve the issue immediately. However, if the CAC is not satisfied that a majority of the workers in the bargaining unit are union members then a secret ballot is held. Where the union can show that 50% of the workers within that bargaining unit are members, the CAC can still order a secret ballot. This would be in circumstances where the CAC believed that a significant number of the trade union members did not want the union to conduct collective bargaining on their behalf or if evidence is produced to this effect. Such evidence would include the circumstances in which employees became or were persuaded to become trade union members and the length of time for which employees have been members of the trade union.

Once a ballot has been ordered the employer must:

- co-operate with the unions in conducting the ballot
- give the union reasonable access to the workers in the bargaining unit
- give CAC the names and addressees of those workers in the bargaining unit and inform CAC when workers leave or join the bargaining unit.

The cost of the ballot is shared equally between the employer and the trade union.

The union can win the ballot, and thus the right to be recognised, only if it is supported by at least 40% of the workers in the bargaining unit and a majority of the workers who vote.

To hold a ballot and persuade workers to vote, the trade union needs access to staff which ensures that whatever resources and channels an employer uses to persuade its employees not to vote for recognition, those same resources are made available to the trade union. A Code of Practice on this point is being produced.

If the union 'wins' recognition and the employer makes no effort to agree how it will collectively bargain with the union, then the CAC will become involved again. It will issue another 'negotiation period' of 30 days or longer, during which time the employer and trade union, with the assistance of the CAC, aim to reach an agreement on a method by which they will conduct collective bargaining. If there is still no agreement then the CAC will issue a final period, known as the Agreement Period, of 20 days or longer. Again the CAC will help both parties to reach an agreement. If there is still no agreement after this period the CAC will specify and impose the method by which the two parties will conduct collective bargaining.

If the union 'loses' the ballot, that trade union is precluded from approaching the employer for three years. Trade unions therefore probably will only target those organisations where they already have 50% membership or where they are likely to win a ballot. Conversely, once recognised, an employer cannot apply to 'de-recognise' the trade union for three years.

It can be seen from these procedures that this is a lengthy and somewhat bureaucratic process. Indeed it is estimated that this detailed procedure, which has to be followed if the employer does not give recognition voluntarily, will take a minimum of six months to complete.

Clearly, making a trade union, particularly one with majority support from the staff, go through this full procedure before gaining recognition will do little to help industrial relations.

Other legislation

The Public Interest Disclosure Act 1999 (otherwise known as the 'Whistle-Blowing' Act)

It is often employees within an organisation who are the first to detect serious irregularities or dangers at work. Yet this information may be kept secret for fear of dismissal or some form of disciplinary action or punishment. Clinical incompetence and medical negligence are examples where the 'offender's' work colleagues are usually the first to notice that something is wrong. In the health world, the Bristol Royal Infirmary and the Rodney Ledward cases in recent years illustrate this point.

Other dramatic examples can be found in the Piper Alpha oil platform explosion and the sinking of the Herald of Free Enterprise cross-channel ferry. The public enquiries held after both these disasters demonstrated that employees of both companies had serious concerns regarding the safety procedures of both vessels prior to the disasters. If those employees had been provided with an internal channel of communication in which to express their concerns without fear of retribution (dismissal or disciplinary action), lives might have been saved.

The aim of the Act is to ensure that employers set up such 'safe' channels. The Act encourages internal disclosure and there are strict definitions as to what types of disclosure will attract protection under the Act.

As with much recent employment law there is a blurring of the definition of the words 'worker' and 'employee'. This Act protects not only employees and ex-employees but those providing direct services to an organisation, e.g. temps from an agency. However, it does not include self-employed contractors.

What is whistle blowing?

The term is used to describe a situation where any worker or ex-worker publicly exposes wrongdoings within an organisation. This can include:

- fraud
- financial mismanagement
- miscarriage of justice
- failure to comply with any legal obligation to which s/he is subject
- breach of health and safety or any other danger
- environmental damage.

In addition, the Act covers information on any matter relating to the above categories that has been, is being or is likely to be deliberately concealed. Box 5.5 summarises these situations.

Box 5.5: Situations covered by the Public Interest Disclosure Act 1999

- criminal offence
- legal obligation
- miscarriage of justice
- health and safety endangered
- environment damaged
- deliberate concealment

It covers acts (or omissions) that have occurred and also those that are occurring and those likely to occur under the above headings.

This Act came into force in July 1999. Before then, employees were extremely exposed if they wished to 'whistle blow' their employers because any such disclosure would be likely to be in breach of an employee's express or implied duty of trust and confidence (see Chapter 2), thereby running the risk of dismissal or disciplinary action.

Under the Act, workers can only claim protection if they are acting in good faith throughout (for example, evidence of any personal benefit from such disclosure would cancel out the good faith protection) and the worker must reasonably believe that the information to be disclosed is substantially true. Acting merely on hearsay or gossip would deprive the worker of protection, as such flimsy sources would contradict any assertions that the worker believed the allegations to be substantially true.

The employee must follow certain procedures in order to gain protection. The intention is for the worker first to go through the organisation's internal channels, for example either the organisation's own whistle blower's procedure or, in the absence of such a procedure, the organisation's grievance procedure. The worker can also go to a prescribed person who will normally be a regulator of the industry, e.g. the GMC for the medical profession or the Health and Safety Executive in relation to health and safety. Disclosure is also protected where it is made to a legal advisor or where the person is employed by a government department or body such as an NHS Trust.

If that fails to resolve the problem or if the employee reasonably believes that the evidence will be destroyed or he or she will suffer a detriment as a result, then disclosure can be made to a third party.

To gain protection in these circumstances, the employee must ensure that they do not make the disclosure for purposes of financial gain and the disclosure must be reasonable in all the circumstances. Contacting the press and being paid to dish the dirt is not what the Act seeks to protect!

Dismissal or detriment suffered as a result of a protected disclosure is unlawful and automatically unfair, irrespective of length of service, and unlimited damages can be awarded.

Clearly, in light of this Act, practices should introduce a whistle-blowing procedure to deal with such issues and to prevent staff disclosing information and then claiming that they did not know what else they could do.

Introducing a whistle blower's procedure

Whistle-blowing procedures should be kept quite separate from a practice's normal grievance procedure as they deal with quite different types of complaint. Grievance procedures address complaints relating to an individual employee, while whistle-blowing complaints affect the organisation as a whole and not necessarily the individual raising the complaints.

While the Act does not require employers to adopt a whistle-blowing policy, there are nevertheless good reasons for implementing such a policy as set out in Box 5.6.

Box 5.6: Benefits of a whistle-blowing policy

- employers are less likely to be exposed to claims at a tribunal since they will be able to demonstrate that they have taken measures to address the concerns of employees
- it is less likely that a public disclosure will be protected
- the existence of the policy may help management identify malpractice before serious harm is caused to the organisation

When designing, introducing and implementing a whistle-blowing policy the following principles need to be considered.

First, the role of management needs to be clear and com-municated to all. Management needs to demonstrate to staff that it expects concerns about malpractice to be raised and that employees, following the whistle-blowing procedure, will have its support. In general practice, partners are often reluctant to raise concerns they may have about another partner's medical practice or behaviour, which can be detrimental to patient safety.

Example 5.2

In a three-partner country practice, two partners began to notice that the middle partner was starting his morning surgeries later and later. He looked heavy-eyed and tired every morning. When they asked after his health his response was very curt and gave the clear impression that he did not wish to discuss the subject. One partner wanted to leave the issue alone, but staff began to notice that the sick partner was for-getting to write up patients' notes. The senior partner raised the issue with the practice manager and she confirmed his observations. She also said that she had overheard one of the staff saying that they had found the sick partner asleep in his consulting room on two occasions when they had arrived early to open up the surgery. There had been a strong smell of alcohol.

The two partners decided to seek advice from the local medical committee (LMC) sick doctor scheme, and also to share with key staff their concerns, from which they learned of more worrying and serious instances of alcohol abuse. They told the sick partner that they wanted him to take leave while seeking help and he did so. The staff were relieved not only about the outcome, but because they had been able to reveal their concerns (in a safe environment) and were taken seriously.

This example shows how important it is that the partners of a practice demonstrate an openness in addressing issues which give cause for concern. It is not possible to reassure staff that the organisation will support concerns about malpractice or dangerous practice if the partners themselves are fearful of raising such issues.

Second, as with many new initiatives, the formation of a working group or other consultation body is helpful in identifying the issues that are important to the organisation, where the risks lie, factors which deter staff from raising concerns and how the whistle-blowing procedures will be implemented.

Third, a whistle-blowing policy must be clear about the type of concerns that should be raised. It is important to make clear that the whistle-blowing procedure is different from the normal grievance procedure and there is no burden on an employee to actually prove the malpractice of which he or she complains. However, it should be made clear that evidence to support the employee's assertion, that they believe their allegations or complaints to be substantially true, will be requested. This prevents flimsy complaints arising from gossip, hearsay or malice.

Fourth, the procedure for responding to complaints needs to be clear and offer whistle blowers confidentiality at the outset. The whistle blower may want to remain anonymous or may insist that his or her name is not disclosed. The procedure should be clear that disclosures of this sort will not be made without the whistle blower's consent. It is important that employees understand what will happen if they make disclosures and that they trust the policy and have confidence in it.

The employer also needs to decide on the appropriate action to be taken in response to a whistle-blowing incident and how the action will be co-ordinated and recorded. The employer may be expected to account to others outside the organisation for the way the matter has been handled. It is also important that feedback is given to the whistle blower so that he or she and other employees are not deterred from using the procedure in future.

To be effective, a whistle-blowing policy should be promoted within the workplace and the level of awareness raised in an appropriate way. Also, once implemented, the policy will need to be properly monitored to check that it is achieving the objectives. Adequate records must be kept of all whistle-blowing incidents and a record kept of how concerns were handled and the outcome of any investigation.

Consulting employee representatives when redundancies are proposed – the Collective Redundancies and Transfer of Undertakings (Protection of Employment) (Amendment) Regulations 1999

These regulations came into effect on 1 November 1999 and they are relevant when it is proposed to make 20 employees redundant at any one time. As this would rarely occur in general practice, the Regulations are not detailed here except to say that at the moment employers making 20 or more staff redundant, and where there is no recognised trade union, are obliged to consult formally with employee representatives. Until these regulations came into force there was no guidance as to how these representatives were to be elected and consulted. The Regulations now specify such procedures.

Equal rights for part-time staff

Until the implementation of the Part-time Workers Directive in April 2000, part-time workers who wished to claim equal access to the same terms and conditions of employment as their full-time colleagues had to use the law on indirect sex discrimination to prove a claim. However, claims for parity can now be made using the more straightforward route of the above Directive. This makes it illegal to discriminate against employees on the grounds of their part-time status. A clear example of such discrimination would be paying a part-time receptionist a lower hourly rate than a full-time receptionist doing the same job. Similarly, selecting staff for redundancy on the grounds of their part-time status would be a clear breach of the law.

As a majority of staff employed in general practice are part time, it is important that all terms and conditions are scrutinised to ensure parity in terms and conditions of employment, including access to training and other benefits.

Chapter 6 continues this theme of the treatment of people in employment with a close look at the sophisticated management skills needed to help people in their professional development and training.

6
Day-to-day people management

We have discussed so far the legal context within which managers manage staff. We now turn to the day-to-day management of employees. This chapter addresses how to get the most out of the team and ways of dealing with problematic staff. Chapter 7 confronts the more intransigent issues of incapability, both performance- and health-related.

One of the biggest challenges for any manager is managing the whole person – developing skills, ownership and fostering creativity. This is often a neglected area of staff management as the ambiguity that commonly surrounds the managing of people is daunting compared to, for example, managing quality via statistical processes or technology via the purchase of new equipment.

It is undeniable that people are unpredictable and their needs are diverse. Such needs may change as they progress through their career and life. Effective management demands a recognition that when people decide to resign from a job because they are unhappy they are often leaving because of other people (frequently their manager) and not necessarily because of the organisation.

It is important to help prevent this and maximise the potential for managers to manage in a way that optimises the chances of retaining staff. Therefore this chapter looks at developing a caring and firm management style and helping staff to achieve their full potential through the active development and training of staff in the knowledge, skills and aptitudes needed both to do their jobs effectively and derive real satisfaction from work.

Caring for staff

The main focus of primary healthcare is to care for patients. What sometimes gets forgotten is the need to care for staff. All of the primary healthcare team have a direct and indirect impact on the quality of care patients receive. It does not start and finish in the consulting or treatment rooms. Caring for members of the team, both individually and collectively, is, therefore, fundamental to ensuring that patients receive the highest possible care from the very beginning of their contact with a practice to the completion of the treatment received.

Example 6.1

A large, busy practice found it was losing patients to a neighbouring practice. The partners instructed the practice manager to research the reasons behind the haemorrhage. She used a number of methods, including a patient satisfaction survey and contacting those patients who had re-registered with the neighbouring surgery. Her findings were startling. Some of the current and past patients identified the length of time they had to wait to see the one female partner as the main cause of dissatisfaction. However, the vast majority of respondents cited the unfriendly atmosphere in reception and the unhelpful and even hostile attitude by many of the receptionists to patients.

The partners were quick to blame the reception staff, but the manager was aware that, due to her own workload, she had failed to undertake many of her key staff management duties. Staff meetings had been cancelled over the past year, the appraisal scheme had fallen into disuse and very little training or staff development was taking place. After consulting with the staff as to their needs, she realised that they felt neglected. She also found out that an adulterous affair between two of the partners was now common knowledge amongst the staff and was contributing significantly to low morale and poor performance.

> With this knowledge and insight she started to improve morale and thus the atmosphere in reception through restoring staff meetings, resurrecting the appraisal scheme, and developing a programme of staff training and education. Armed with her findings, she managed to get the senior partner to confront the partners' affair and one of them eventually left the practice.

The duty to care for practice staff has legal, managerial and moral implications. The concept of caring for employees (the duty of care) arises from the need for employers to exercise power with responsibility. Obviously, 'caring' is about more than simply exercising one's legal responsibilities, and practices frequently focus on fostering a 'family' atmosphere. However, it must always be remembered that as employers, practices have the right, ultimately, to terminate staff contracts. This tension, which exists in all contracts of employment – the imbalance in the power between the two parties to the contract – can be forgotten by doctors, who often expect staff to operate and behave as if there is an equal relationship between employer and employee. The real impact is that staff will not necessarily speak freely and openly about their professional needs, or raise grievances, unless they have some form of safe structure within which to test the water of an employer's tolerance to criticism. Staff will resort to deception if they perceive that their employment may be at risk. As Example 6.2 shows, if staff are unclear about the practice's attitude to time off when childcare arrangements break down, employees in this situation will phone in sick to get the time off work.

Example 6.2

Megan was a practice nurse with three months' service at the practice. When she started, she was given a six-month probationary period. Megan was a single parent with a 3-year-old daughter, Bunty. She had an arrangement with her neighbour Joan to collect Bunty from nursery each day until she came home from work. This worked well until Megan and Joan quarrelled and Joan refused to continue looking after Bunty.

Feeling anxious that she would fail her probationary period if she took time off work to look after Bunty and, for the same reason, not wanting to ask for a short period of reduced hours, Megan tried all sorts of ruses to cope while she desperately looked for a replacement for Joan. She started slipping out of the treatment room to collect Bunty and bringing her to the practice 'so everyone could see her'. She persuaded the nursery to keep Bunty late for two days and she went sick on another day.

After a week of this behaviour the practice manager asked what was going on and Megan broke down in tears and told her of her problem. The practice manager reassured her that not only did Megan have a legal right to some time off to make arrangements for Bunty's care, but also the practice was very sympathetic to this sort of problem. They discussed ways of resolving the issue, which included Megan leaving work early for the next week to collect Bunty, and meanwhile a nanny employed by one of the partners put Megan in touch with a recommended child-minder, who proved most suitable. Megan was able to resume her full-time hours knowing that she was working with a highly supportive team and a caring employer.

The duty of care also means caring about standards of performance and conduct. Tolerating sloppy work or unacceptable behaviour is not about being 'nice'. It demonstrates a lack of care for the individual concerned by allowing them to perform inadequately, and also for the other team members who can soon start to feel demotivated and even resentful if the practice fails to address issues of unacceptable standards of work or conduct. General practitioners and practice managers need themselves to demonstrate and model the sort of conduct and care for others that they expect of staff. In addition, managers in primary care actively need to design systems, procedures and processes that enable staff to operate in an open and honest way, actively contributing to the organisation, where they are able to achieve their very best.

At the very minimum, practices need to have the employment policies and procedures set out in Box 6.1.

Box 6.1: Employment policies and procedures

- **a health and safety policy**, which is understood and applied by all members of the team
- **an equal opportunities policy**, which includes a commitment to the appointment, promotion and training of staff free of illegal discrimination, and what to do in cases of allegations of harassment and bullying (see Appendices A and B)
- **a grievance procedure and a disciplinary procedure**, which follows the ACAS Codes of Practice on Disciplinary and Grievance Procedures in Employment (see Appendices D, E and F)
- **sickness and long-term absence procedures**, which balance the needs of the individual with the needs of the practice. (see Chapter 7)

The above are just some of the policies many practices will have in place in one form or another. It is important to remember that fulfilling the employer's responsibility of care to employees is also very much about common sense and 'do as one would be done by'. The ability to empathise is a much under-rated but essential attribute in anyone who is responsible for staff, both in exercising one's duty of care and in the general management, development and motivation of people, as Example 6.3 shows.

Example 6.3

The partners of a practice were frustrated with the poor performance of their practice manager and tried to resolve the problem through gradually taking over many of her managerial duties. This was done in a piecemeal fashion and she was told on each occasion that the reason behind the transfer of responsibilities was that she was obviously overworked. The manager felt patronised and, with each erosion of her responsibilities, her feelings of insecurity and stress increased. She eventually went on long-term sick with depression.

> It was only when one of her close colleagues at work, the practice nurse, asked the partners to put themselves in the manager's shoes that they recognised that their failure to empathise had led them to behave in a thoughtless and careless fashion. What had been a tricky but manageable performance issue had now developed into a long-term issue and a far more difficult problem to resolve.

In addition, some recent research has for the first time demonstrated that actively managing people in a considered and professional way has a direct effect on the success of an organisation.

The Institute of Work Psychology, University of Sheffield (West and Patterson 1998), undertook research into identifying the factors that most contributed to organisational profit and productivity. The research involved 100 employers over a seven-year period. It revealed that the development of people is not only critical to business performance but it also far outstrips emphasis on quality, technology, competitive strategy or research and development in its influence on profitability.

Although the research was undertaken in the business community, it holds findings of interest to all organisations that employ people and are curious as to the factors which contribute to organisational success. The research demonstrates that employees' skills are best acquired by effective recruitment and selection, that those skills are best enhanced by strategic training and appraisals, and that people are best employed in jobs designed to promote employee autonomy, flexibility and problem solving.

Specifically, the research reveals that there are two forms of personnel management practice related to organisational success. They are:

- the acquisition and development of skills (as assessed by the sophistication of induction training, selection and appraisal practices)
- job design (as assessed by the degree of job variety, responsibility, skill flexibility and teamwork).

West and Patterson were able to quantify the percentage difference in variances in profitability of different factors. The results are surprising:

- research and development   8%
- people management (as defined above)   19%
- quality, new technology and competitive strategy   1%.

The research goes on to demonstrate that not only are people unpredictable and their needs diverse but organisational success depends on management's ability to respond to such diversity. One of the most effective tools for managing this diversity and helping people achieve their potential is regular appraisal interviews conducted by appraisers trained in this most skilful and demanding of personnel management activities.

This chapter therefore identifies specifically and addresses the importance of appraisal, conducting a staff appraisal interview and, coupled with this, the role that training and development play in modern primary healthcare.

Appraisal

The performance of the whole practice is high on the current primary healthcare agenda. Given this focus on quality performance, together with the introduction of clinical governance and revalidation, it is not surprising that appraisal is becoming one of the most popular management tools being introduced into primary healthcare. Indeed both the management-led clinical governance and the professional-led revalidation have appraisal at their cores.

The GMC's (2000) initiative to introduce revalidation for doctors has specifically stated that a basic element for revalidation will be regular, formative appraisal. Appraisals are the cornerstone of the proposed revalidation procedures for all doctors (Irvine 1999). Stage 1 of the procedure will be a doctor's profile – data based on showing:

- a record of professional educational activity
- a portfolio of wider professional development
- a record of participation in and results of clinical and organisational audit
- the results of regular appraisals which should reflect the above, showing any changes in the doctor's performance and set in the context of national professional standards.

Clinical governance proposals and their complementary proposals set out in *Supporting Doctors, Protecting Patients* (Chief Medical Officer 1999) lay great emphasis on the identification of poor performance. A system of 'annual appraisal', including an assessment of clinical standards, is proposed to ensure that this is done.

It is clear therefore that the drive towards appraisal as a legitimate management tool has expanded from 'management' to clinicians. Practices will need to become involved in appraisal for both doctors and staff. It will become a fundamental area of clinical and practice management in the future. Many practices have already embraced appraisal in a variety of forms. In addition to the traditional format of employer appraising employee, some practices now have group appraisal using 'significant events' as a tool to examine and discuss performance. There is also peer review where each partner is appraised by others in the practice. Peer appraisal in the vocational training scheme setting is also gaining popularity.

The North of England Region of vocational training for GPs has already introduced a system of appraisal for trainers by associate directors (Haman and Irvine 1998) and the North East Scotland Region is currently designing a system of peer appraisal of trainers.

Introducing an appraisal scheme is predicated on the recognition that the development of an individual can be best addressed by the use of an effective appraisal system, which of itself should be the central plank of any practice's quality control arrangements (Irvine and Haman 1997). This opportunity to have protected time to consider, analyse and discuss one's own performance and development needs can be beneficial to both the individual and the practice.

Nevertheless, the word 'appraisal' conjures up for most people the concepts of judgement and criticism. We know from our own experiences that a person's sense of self-worth and value are deeply invested in their own and others' perceptions of their job performance. When this area of one's life comes under scrutiny, then even the most self-confident will experience some form of anxiety.

Managing this anxiety and ensuring that the outcome of the appraisal interview, during, immediately after and in the long term, is constructive for the individuals concerned and the practice is not easy. Indeed, it could be argued that an appraisal interview is probably one of the most sophisticated types of interview managers have to conduct. The need therefore for effective and sophisticated training and the opportunity to practise appraisal interviewing techniques is obvious.

If the value statements inherent in the introduction of an effective performance appraisal scheme are clear and agreed beforehand, the benefit will be greater. Such value statements could include the following:

- a recognition that people are the most important constituent of any organisation and that employees do not necessarily develop automatically but need to be cultivated and developed in a planned and consistent fashion
- in general practice, high performance depends crucially on attending to people's developmental needs
- each person in the practice is entitled to have access to and be given the opportunity to discuss information about his or her performance, skills and achievements, and to know how these are evaluated.

An outline of an appraisal interview is now described.

An appraisal interview

Preparation

It is essential in any appraisal interview that the appraisee has confidence in the integrity of the appraiser. This is even more important when dealing with problematic staff. Ensuring that such sensitive issues are handled constructively and assertively requires thorough preparation beforehand. If the interview is to be well-balanced and non-personal, collecting examples of both good and poor performance over the appraisal period is essential. Timing is important in this preparatory activity. It is easy to focus on the past few weeks and ignore performance over the whole year. Many people receive two-week rather than annual appraisals because of this tendency by appraisers to restrict the scope of this preparatory work to the recent past.

Opening the interview

The first aim is to relax the appraisee as he or she must be able to make full use of this opportunity to reflect objectively on successes and failures. The competence of the appraiser as a willing mentor is crucial to this process. Establishing rapport and allowing the appraisee both to reflect on past performance and express their hopes and plans for the future is fundamental to the interview's success.

To enable the appraisee to appraise himself or herself and to suggest ways of improving or building on current strengths and interests, do remember that individuals are far more committed to a line of action if they themselves have suggested it. The interview therefore should be not be focused on the appraiser telling but rather encouraging the appraisee to assess his or her own strengths and weaknesses and to come up with ideas to improve performance and identify development needs.

Tackling problems

Appraisal interviews can be emotional minefields. Even so there is no excuse for not tackling areas of under performance or fudging sensitive issues. Indeed failing to do so will adversely affect the credibility of the appraisal scheme.

Concentrate on performance and not on personality. If the appraisee, for example, is abrupt with patients, give instances where this has happened, describing only the behaviour and deliver this in a calm, non-judgemental voice. Ask for views and refrain from labelling the appraisee as rude or abrupt. There is little you can do about an individual's personality. What you can do is change behaviour and that is the issue to address.

Make your assertions clear and unambiguous and supported by facts, not feelings.

Closing the interview

Agree targets and objectives with timescales and follow-up dates. If appropriate, ask the appraisee to summarise the main points of the interview. This can reinforce commitment to change and helps to ascertain the depth and accuracy of the appraisee's understanding of the issues discussed.

While discussing training and development needs, ensure that false expectations are not raised. It is easy to imply that a person will receive training and education, which may not be feasible.

Individual and practice performance will be enhanced if information and knowledge are available, assessed objectively and discussed skilfully. Time spent attending to individual performance yields demonstrable benefits to the practice, the individual and the appraiser's management skills and competence.

The importance of this tool, when it is used with expertise, cannot be overemphasised. But its introduction needs careful preparation. Poor appraisals have the potential to diminish, demotivate and alienate staff.

Training and development

Identifying the professional needs of staff is a fundamental aim of most appraisal schemes and, as can be seen from the previous section, the concept of professional development has infiltrated the whole of the medical profession. Doctors qualifying after their initial training and continuing to practise with no further assessment will be a thing of the past. The importance of training and development has shifted from the didactic to the facilitative, with individuals taking more responsibility for their own learning and development.

Generally, training remains a much underinvested activity in the UK. Its importance can be summed up by The Body Shop advert 'If you think education is expensive, try ignorance'. This view is amply born out by all organisations that have been faced with problems caused by undertrained staff. After all, part of the implied terms of any contract of employment is to ensure staff are appropriately skilled to do the tasks asked of them.

A useful starting point, therefore, to changing the practice's attitude (and therefore investment of money and time) to training and development is to assess its organisational approach to staff development. Cunningham (1994) identified four types of organisations in relation to training and development, set out in Box 6.2. This shows that in strategic organisations, managers see their roles as developers and leaders. They question and encourage others and handle mistakes as opportunities to learn.

Cunningham's analysis is reflected in the view, held by experts in the field of developing staff, that in order to meet the sophisticated needs of today's workforce, trainers must:

- cease acting as transmitters of knowledge and instead become development advisers
- become mentors, facilitators, guides and coaches
- be better at listening than presenting, capable of drawing out contributions rather than delivering the latest word.

Box 6.2: Organisational types in terms of training and development

---

Apathetic/antagonistic organisations have the following characteristics:
- do not care about employee development or are even actively opposed to learning
- fear losing staff to competitors

Reactive organisations have the following characteristics:
- are prepared to support people's development
- staff have to pester the boss for training
- focus is tactical (to solve an immediate problem)
- little or no planning
- no coherent training strategy

Bureaucratic organisations have the following characteristics:
- substantial investment
- standardised courses not geared to the individual's career needs or strategic needs of the organisation
- empty gestures
- low expectations that the training will change people

Strategic organisations have the following characteristics:
- public commitment to learning, supported by top management
- continued learning is fundamental to the business strategy
- avoid using the term 'human resources'
- collaborate with the individual's career strategies

But they must be experts on how people learn and skilled in delivering a variety of ways to achieve this.

Personal development and its linked concepts, continuous professional development and career management, are becoming increasingly important to individuals. The breakdown of the 'job-for-life' approach to work has meant that, in order to maximise their employability, people need to develop their potential and continue to learn throughout life. Wise organisations recognise this and provide opportunities for their employees to experience, reflect and grow, not always just within the requirements of their job or indeed their organisation, but often more widely. However, many organisations, including general practice, tend to be a combination of Cunningham's types – the reactive organisation with some characteristics of the bureaucratic.

It follows therefore that in order to become a more strategic organisation, practices need to embrace strategic rather than reactive training, personal development plans (PDPs) and continuous professional development (CPD). Strategic training and the initiatives of PDP and CPD all fit and reflect this move away from the didactic to the facilitative. Let us look at these in more detail.

Strategic training

Any training activity should ideally be part of an integrated strategic planning process. This is what is meant by the term 'strategic training'. When changes occur within organisations, if training comes as an afterthought it will be reactive and almost certainly less effective than strategic training. Training plans need to be designed within the context of all stages in the training process, i.e. assessment, design, delivery and evaluation. Each stage should have a subplan, which clearly sets out the objectives and provides a guide for action and measurement.

Continuous professional development (CPD) and personal development plans (PDPs)

The rest of this chapter addresses PDPs and CPD. The terms CPD and PDP can become interchangeable and, as a result, confusing. The differences between them are mainly in emphasis. CPD can be seen as driven by professional institutions to ensure up-to-date knowledge; PDPs as being driven by the individual to meet personal goals. They are both concerned with enabling individuals to grow and realise their potential.

Continuous professional development

Continuous professional development affects members of professions whose institutes control qualification and practise registration. Most now apply systems of CPD, which require members of that profession to demonstrate evidence that their skills and knowledge are being updated and maintained. CPD is based on the premise that professionals need to update their knowledge and skills continuously. The primary responsibility lies with the individual; however, employers are often asked to pay for the training element of CPD and certain aspects of CPD may be covered by internal work experience.

Marples (1999) has written that for the purposes of CPD, learning is assumed to be derived from four main sources:

1 learning from the workplace, e.g. managing change, adoption of best practice, meeting unusual or challenging objectives, leading a major project
2 learning from structured sources, e.g. conferences, courses, distance learning material
3 learning from self-directed personal work, e.g. reading of 'learned journals', library work, research
4 learning from other environments that transfer into one's working life, e.g. voluntary work, public office, giving talks.

These are not mutually exclusive areas. There is a need to keep a record of personal learning against these headings and it is proposed that members of the Institute of Healthcare Management (IHM) would acquire 20 points a year or, for a longer course of study, 60 points over three years. Attendance at an IHM day event may qualify for 10 points, with routine reading of journals qualifying for a maximum of five points. A particularly demanding set of organisational objectives that requires new ideas might meet the full 20 points.

Primary care clinicians as well as managers are also in the vanguard of CPD and PDP. The Royal College of General

Practitioners (RCGP 1999) has stated that the current system of continuing medical education (CME) is flawed as it encourages education for its own sake without first identifying educational needs. It is hoped that CPD − the evidence of which will be contained in each doctor's PDP − will ensure that educational needs are identified and met with a change to clinical practice, demonstrating improvements in patient care.

Personal development plans

Despite its name, a PDP is an organisational tool. An employee needs support to develop his or her PDP and, linked with appraisals, PDPs can focus on the current job, development for the next job or the person's overall effectiveness.

For employees, PDPs start with the individual's current post. Asking employees to analyse their day-to-day tasks and how they manage them can lead to the development of a learning plan. Such a plan would include how and when this learning will be achieved and how it will be reviewed. To get the maximum benefit from PDPs, employees need to keep a learning log, which records the process and identifies the methods of learning used. These are detailed in Box 6.3 and share many of the methods listed for CPD by Marples.

Box 6.3: Methods of learning

Structured	Semi-structured or unstructured
Training courses	Coaching
Job swap	Counselling
Distance learning	Mentoring
Development centres	Discussion
Appraisals	Observation
Developmental work assignments	Reading
Facilitated learning reviews	Keeping a journal
Working towards NVQ/FBA or other	Networking
accreditation	Voluntary/community work

Fostering a climate of trust and mutual respect is important if employees are to discuss fully their personal development needs with their managers. Similarly, GPs and registrars need to feel they are engaging with others who are supportive rather than judgemental when discussing their PDPs with colleagues. This argues for a practice- and profession-wide approach to personal development, so that everyone is in the same position, experiencing and defining PDPs in the same way. Some practices have integrated the design of PDPs with practice development plans (Elwyn and Smail 1998). This really does incorporate a strategic training approach into PDPs.

The most crucial aspect of personal development is that people must be self-reliant and own their PDP. Interventions from others need to be facilitative rather than prescriptive or controlling. In any sample of employees, however, a minority will not have the motivation to develop themselves. This may be difficult to accept, but there are limits to how far employees can be expected to pursue personal development activities where they can see no benefit to themselves. For example, a receptionist with 25 years' experience and in her retirement year may be less motivated to participate in a PDP than a younger practice administrator just embarking on a career in primary care management.

There is a potential problem in that some staff may see personal development as leading to promotion. There is not necessarily any connection between the two and this must be explained at the outset to avoid later disappointment. This is particularly relevant to general practice, where opportunities within a practice will be limited due to the size of the organisation.

It may also be necessary to clarify which personal development activities the organisation can support. For example, supporting development that helps the employee undertake their current or expected job requirements would be a natural function for the practice, with perhaps partial support for broader development that is not directly related to the person's job. For example, it may emerge from an appraisal interview that the practice manager needs training in new technological developments, which will progress his/her job and benefit the practice. Additional personal developmental needs identified may include a postgraduate management qualification, which may not directly benefit the practice but will develop the manager and give her greater career potential. The practice in this example may decide fully to support the first need and support the second developmental need through allowing day-release with 50% funding of fees.

The benefits of PDPs are many and various. Developing an organisational culture which values personal development brings benefits to everyone. Employees who take a mature approach to their personal development welcome the responsibility and will provide the organisation with a broader and deeper understanding of their capabilities and potential.

When a problem in the performance of an individual is identified, one of the first interventions is usually to offer some form of training to improve matters. However, training will not always improve matters or may even be an inappropriate reaction to the problem. Chapter 7 addresses issues of capability that require a more complex and often subtle response.

7
Capability issues

It is a fact of life that even with best management in the world there will always be situations where employees seem incapable of doing their jobs to the standard expected by the organisation. Also, people do fall ill, sometimes for long periods of time, causing them to be incapable on physical or mental grounds of undertaking their jobs. Both these situations are catered for in employment law, allowing the employer legally to address the problem and, in some cases, eventually dismiss the employee.

The legal definition of capability at work can be found in The Employment Rights Act 1996:

> capability assessed by reference to skill, aptitude, health or any other physical or mental quality which relates to work of the kind which the employee was employed to do.

This chapter looks at these two aspects of capability – health, encompassing the whole area of absence management, and skill or aptitude.

Absences in the practice

Many managers treat sickness absence of staff as an act of God, something that has to be tolerated and endured rather than a management or organisational issue that can be addressed actively. Effective management of absence requires, above all, an active, not a passive approach, and it often involves balancing the needs of the employee with the needs of the practice. Managers need to distinguish between long-term absence caused by acute or chronic illness and persistent or frequent short-term absences caused by unconnected minor ailments, as each raises particular issues. For example, a known chronic illness necessitating outpatient appointments or a forthcoming elective operation are conditions which lend themselves to planning beforehand, with cover for the absentee arranged in advance. In contrast to this, the employee who regularly takes single days off sick for unrelated illnesses demands cover arranged in haste with other staff working overtime and a deterioration in the service offered to patients.

The legal context of absence is clear. Staff have a contractual obligation to work the days and hours stated in their contract of employment except where the contract allows them time off work. These permissible periods of absence, most commonly holidays and sick leave, usually carry with them rules, which the employee must follow for the absence to be authorised and, if relevant, to receive a salary or proportion thereof, during the period of the absence.

As in any other management situation, the starting point for good management of absence is to ensure that all staff are aware of their contractual obligations. The information given to employees, usually through the statement of terms and conditions of employment, must detail the procedures to be used when they are absent from work. Indeed, ensuring that comprehensive and clear rules and procedures are communicated to staff provides the framework within which problematic absences are managed. Although this sounds obvious, many organisations have such vague rules that both managers and staff have difficulty in applying them consistently and it makes dealing with problematic absences very difficult.

Box 7.1 sets out some questions to consider when reviewing the contract of employment and the rules relating to absence. The questions cover holiday leave, sickness absence, long-term ill health and other special leave.

Box 7.1: Questions to consider when reviewing the contract of employment and the rules relating to absence

---

Holiday leave
Do the rules relating to holiday leave specify:
- how the leave is calculated?
- the process of arranging the leave and with whom?
- the criteria to be used as to who gets priority when holiday leave requests clash?
- what can happen if the rules are not followed?

Sick leave
Similarly with sickness absence, do the rules specify:
- that staff are not allowed to register as patients of the practice?
- by when and to whom the employee is to make contact on the first day of absence?
- when self and medical certificates are required?
- the maximum number of days in any one 'sick year' that can be covered by self-certification?
- that sickness absences are monitored and that frequent sickness absences may give rise to formal discussions with the practice manager?
- that the disciplinary procedure may eventually be applied when staff exceed the permitted number of days absence in any one period?

Long-term sickness
Do the rules specify:
- the right of the practice to request a medical examination of the employee and to receive medical reports?
- that a senior member of the practice will keep in regular contact with the employee including visiting him or her at home?
- the period of time after which the practice may consider terminating employment?

Other leave
Do the terms of employment specify:
- the events which give rise to special leave, e.g. bereavement, public duties?
- the person to whom such requests should be made and the process?

Unauthorised absence

Should a member of staff suddenly fail to appear for work without contacting the practice, it is important that action is taken promptly and fairly in dealing with the situation.

The first step is to attempt to contact the employee during the first day of absence; this also gives the message to other staff that attendance at work is important and that absences will be dealt with promptly. If telephone calls fail to establish contact then a letter asking him or her to contact the practice immediately on receipt should be sent. Further attempts to telephone should follow, as the employee may indeed be too ill to contact the practice or may be suffering some form of trauma.

If contact cannot be established, a further letter should be sent detailing the employee's contractual obligations and that failure to contact the practice may result in the commencement of disciplinary action. Of course, real life is not as straightforward as this and most practice managers will no doubt know the employee's family or friends, which can help in establishing contact. They will also know the employment history of staff, and the way in which such absences are handled will be determined by whether such incidents have happened before and length of service. A member of staff new to the practice will obviously be treated differently from a long-standing employee with no history of such behaviour.

The golden rule is to behave – and to be seen to behave – professionally and reasonably in a way appropriate to the employee's role, length of service and history. Ultimately, an employee can be dismissed for breach of contract; however, any such dismissal should follow the practice's disciplinary procedure, which itself should follow the ACAS code on discipline (see Chapter 8).

Sickness absence in the practice

In addition to keeping accurate attendance records of staff, there must be clarity in the levels of intermittent absences which will be acceptable before the matter is investigated and ultimately disciplinary action considered. These sickness records need to be monitored and checked regularly so that if an employee attains more than the specified number of days absence within a period, this fact can be identified and acted on. Details of this sort of absence monitoring should be included in the information given to all staff when they commence work with the practice.

There are generally three forms of sickness absence:

- staff who are occasionally ill
- staff who are regularly absent through unrelated illnesses
- staff on long-term sickness.

As far as the first category is concerned, most people fall ill at some point in their lives. Indeed this is recognised by society through the payment of sickness benefits and contracts of employment which allow for absence from work due to sickness or injury. It is the second and third type of absence that can prove problematic.

The regular absentee

This type of employee is often the most difficult to manage. Absences will be covered by self or medical certificates and as they are unexpected and for a short duration, it is very difficult for the practice to plan and manage the absent employee's work.

In managing all sickness absences, but particularly in relation to staff with a poor attendance record, there are a number of good practices to follow. All staff should be told the name of the person to whom they must speak when they first phone in to report their sickness. This person needs to be a supervisor or a manager who has been trained to deal with such phone calls. Staff need to know that leaving a message with a colleague is unacceptable and that if they do so then the manager will telephone them at home.

During this initial contact with the practice, the person designated to receive these calls should ensure that they have a full discussion, if practicable, with the staff member, irrespective of whether the employee is suspected of malingering. These conversations should be conducted in a sympathetic manner. Box 7.2 sets out the types of question it would be appropriate to ask during this conversation.

Box 7.2: Questions to ask when staff phone in sick

- what is wrong? Can you be specific?
- how long do you think you'll be away?
- can the practice do anything to help?
- when will you contact me again?

Example 7.1 illustrates this point.

Example 7.1

One of the nurses in a practice had a poor attendance record with self certificates covering her frequent absences. On the mornings of her absences, when she telephoned the practice, she tended to speak to a nurse colleague who passed on messages to the practice manager giving the reason for her absences. The practice decided to tighten up on their sickness rules and the nurse was now obliged to speak to the practice manager (or in her absence a designated partner). On taking these calls the manager asked all employees who phoned in sick questions similar to those in Box 7.2. Consequently the nurse's attendance record improved and there was an overall decrease, albeit small, in the number of sickness days taken by staff.

When the employee returns to work, the manager/senior receptionist should interview him or her. These 'return-to-work' interviews are time-consuming and may be felt to be unnecessary but they are a very important part of any absence control procedure. They have a number of very useful purposes, which are set out in Box 7.3. Such interviews need to be conducted confidentially and with sensitivity. During the interview the manager needs to discuss the illness and to enquire as to how the person is feeling. Too often, self certificates are not followed up in this way and this can facilitate malingering. A record needs to be kept of the interview. The strong message conveyed through the return-to-work interview is that an absence is a significant, not a minor, event for the practice and means that an important member of the team is missing.

Box 7.3: Purposes of the 'return-to-work' interview

- to help in the monitoring of absence of particular staff
- to act as a deterrent for those employees whose absences are not due to a genuine illness
- to show concern by the employer, particularly in seeking confirmation that the employee is fully recovered
- to enable the identification of a common thread to any intermittent illnesses
- to alert the practice to problems, health or otherwise, staff are experiencing

If a pattern of absences is emerging the employee needs to be seen and his or her attention drawn to the emerging pattern. It is important to try to find out the reasons why so much time has been taken off work. If the cause is work-related, then the practice and the employee can start to address and resolve the problem, as Example 7.2 shows.

Example 7.2

A practice's secretary had started to take a lot of time off work, mainly Mondays. When she was interviewed about the emerging pattern she confided that her marriage was breaking down and her husband had left her and the three children. After a weekend of stress and looking after her young children alone, she often felt she could not face work on a Monday morning. After some negotiation the secretary's hours were changed and her hours were reduced so that she started work at lunchtime on Mondays. It was agreed that the situation from the practice's and her point of view would be reviewed in three months' time.

Where there are a number of people in the practice taking regular days off under the guise of sickness, then the problem needs to be probed at a deeper level and the following questions asked about any common factors:

- does the same person supervise them?
- do they all work closely with one of the partners?
- do they share the same workspace?

One of the most common indicators of low staff morale is high absence figures. If the problem is widespread, then the whole management of the practice and the effect on staff may need to be reviewed. It might be worthwhile comparing the practice's sickness statistics with neighbouring practices of similar size, to assess the extent of the problem.

If there are no underlying issues, often one quiet chat about the pattern of behaviour will be enough to see an improvement in the employee's attendance. If the behaviour continues then consideration should be given to commencing the disciplinary procedure. If the illness is not a chronic condition and the absences are due to unrelated medical complaints it is important to resist referring the employee to a doctor for a medical opinion. All that will result is involving the practice in a medical issue which, by definition (unless related to a mental illness) will throw little light on the problem.

The practice may decide that there is an unacceptable level of short-term persistent absence, which might justify dismissal. In that case, it is essential that a staged warning is implemented before any decision to dismiss takes place and that the employee is treated with sympathy and understanding throughout. The stages of warnings are as follows:

- informal counselling
- verbal warning
- written warning
- final written warning
- formal trial period
- termination of employment
- appeal procedure.

Following any warnings and/or discussions, the employee needs to be given time to improve.

If the employee appears to be suffering a genuine illness, a number of factors need to be considered before any decision to dismiss is taken. These factors include:

- the nature of the illness and the prognosis
- length of absences and intervals of normal attendance at work
- the effects on the practice of the absence
- whether the employee has been regularly consulted about his or her attendance and its potential consequences
- any alternative employment the practice could offer which would be more suitable to the person
- if the employee is protected by the Disability Discrimination Act, any adjustments the practice can make to continue employing him or her (see Chapter 3).

Dismissal for ill health absence will usually be on the grounds of capability. However, if the employer reasonably believes that the illness(s) is not genuine, then dismissal can be on the grounds of misconduct. Chapter 8 deals in detail with disciplinary and dismissal issues.

Long-term sickness

The above procedures for short-term absences – reporting rules, return-to-work interviews – are as valid for long-term absences. However, the following additional factors and procedures need to be borne in mind.

Employers often treat staff on long-term sick leave rather preciously in the mistaken belief that absences covered by medical certificates have some legal protection against intervention. Often the issue of a member of staff on long-term leave is only addressed when he or she is approaching the expiration of their sickness leave entitlement. This can be interpreted as uncaring and can also delay both the practice's ability to manage the absence constructively and the handling of any future termination of employment on grounds of capability. As Example 7.3 illustrates, a reluctance to visit the employee can be counterproductive.

Example 7.3

A practice's manager suffered a stroke and was on long-term sick leave. The partners visited her in hospital and once when she was at home recuperating. The manager duly sent in medical certificates covering her absence but received no further visits. When she was on the brink of exhausting her sick leave entitlement the partners took expensive legal advice on how to dismiss her on grounds of capability and were steeling themselves on how to break the news of the termination of her employment.

However, before any further visit was made they received her letter of resignation. This letter informed them that early on in her illness she had decided that the severity of her condition, the time needed to rehabilitate and the prognosis for her condition would prevent her from resuming her position with the practice. The letter also informed them that she would have liked the opportunity to discuss this decision with them and had assumed, erroneously, that at least one of them would have called to see her on a regular basis. She felt rather abandoned and depressed that her employers had taken so little interest in her.

When an employee is absent due to an illness, which may be long-term, it is important to establish regular contact. Not only does this ensure that the employee is aware that the practice cares about him or her but it also allows the practice to gain information about the nature and extent of the illness, follow progress and hopefully the eventual recovery of the employee. Regular visits will provide information in preparing for the employee's return to work or ways of terminating the employee's employment fairly, sympathetically and legally. For those few employees who exploit their sickness leave entitlement, regular fortnightly or monthly visiting ensures that he or she is aware that the absence is being actively managed and monitored. But also importantly, if an employee cannot return to work he or she may lack the confidence or knowledge as to how to broach the subject. Regular visiting provides the opportunity for discussing the employee's future with the practice and the individual's opinions on his or her illness in the security of their own home.

Regular visiting also gives vital information as to when and from whom – family doctor/specialist, etc. – a medical opinion should be sought. Information about the employee's true medical condition needs to be sought to manage the long-term illness, particularly if dismissal is being considered. Box 7.4 gives an example of the sort of letter that should be sent to the employee seeking permission to gain the information required and, following the Access to Medical Reports Act 1988, setting out the legal requirements. Box 7.5 is an example of a letter which the employee should sign giving that permission.

Box 7.4: Letter to the employee from the employer

Dear [*name of employee*],

Further to my visit on ..., due to the length of time you have now been absent from work through ill health, it is important that I have some idea when you will be fit to return to work.

In order to ascertain this information, I would like to contact your [*GP/specialist/consultant*] as soon as possible. I am only able to contact *him/her* after receiving written permission from yourself to do so. To this end I enclose a letter giving me permission to contact [*name of physician*]. You will see from the enclosure that I have assumed that you will wish to exercise your right to have access to the report. Your rights, under the Medical Reports Act 1988, include:

- access to the medical report before it is sent to me
- comment on and request for amendments to be made to that medical report
- refusing consent for the report to be given to me.

If it is convenient, I would like to visit you again on ...... at .... During this visit we can discuss this letter and the enclosure and any thoughts you may have on the prognosis of your illness. You will receive a copy of the letter I will send to [*GP/specialist/consultant*].

In the meanwhile I wish you a very speedy recovery.

Yours sincerely,

Name of employer

Box 7.5: Letter from employee to employer giving permission to contact the physician and requesting access to the report before it is sent to the employer

Dear [*name of employer*],

I give you permission to contact [*name and address of doctor*] to ascertain a medical report on my current state of health and its prognosis. I also wish to exercise my right to have access to that report before it is sent to you.

Yours sincerely,

Name of employee

The letter from the employee can then be sent to the relevant medical practitioner, duly signed by the employee, with a covering letter as set out in Box 7.6.

Box 7.6: Letter from the employer to the doctor

Dear Doctor....,

Re: [*name of employee*]

[*Name of employee*] is your patient and has been absent from work since ..... *His/her* period of absence has been covered by medical certificates signed by yourself (and/or partners). It is now important that as *his/her* employer we have some information which will help us manage *his/her* absence and arrange the appropriate cover for *his/her* duties.

I am therefore writing to you to ask if you would be able to provide us with a report of [*name of employee*]'s illness, the prognosis and some indication of when *he/she* will be fit to return to work to undertake *his/her* job as [*job title*].

It would also be appreciated if you could provide us with any other relevant information, for example special medication *she/he* may be taking, with any side effects etc. which would be important for *his/her* employers to be aware of prior to *his/her* return to work.

I enclose *his/her* current job description and hours of work. I am also enclosing [*name of employee*]'s letter giving permission for you to provide us with a medical report and exercising *his/her* rights under the Medical Reports Act 1988 to have access to the report etc. prior to it being sent to me.

I would appreciate it if you could advise me of the date you send the report to [*name of employee*] to enable me to monitor the situation and ensure that we receive your report as soon as is practicable. I enclose an s.a.e. for this purpose and look forward to hearing from you soon.

Yours sincerely,

Name of employer
cc Name of employee

While seeking information about the diagnosis and prognosis of the condition, it is important to keep in mind that medical information is only one piece of evidence that a practice needs to take into account. The importance of the post and the ease with which temporary staff can be placed to cover the absence are also relevant factors when looking at and assessing the most appropriate ways of managing long-term sickness. Ultimately it is a management, not a medical, decision that has to be made.

Having maintained regular contact and consulted with the employee, the situation needs to be reviewed and the following options considered:

- employee's eventual return to work
- employee returning to work on revised terms, for example different hours of work or alternative employment; considering these sorts of adjustments are a legal requirement if the employee is protected by the DDA
- terminate employment on grounds of capability.

Chapter 8 deals in detail with the procedure to be used if, on the receipt of this medical information and other evidence, the employer decides to dismiss the employee on grounds of capability.

Poor performance

We now come to the aspect of capability that causes more headaches to managers than almost any other personnel issue – poorly performing staff.

If there is problem with a member of staff, it is important to resist the temptation to reach a quick assessment as to the reasons why someone is performing below standard. Identifying the real problem or underlying causes may take some time.

First, the manager needs to look critically at his or her own management style as this may be a contributory factor. Indeed, it is useful for all people with responsibility for others to examine the way they exercise their management responsibilities. Over- or under-supervising staff can have a detrimental effect on standards of work. An over-supervising manager can be characterised as a person who emphasises 'how' to do things rather than 'what' needs to be done. As a result, employees continually have to prove themselves, new ideas are rejected and the manager has to be 'in control' at all times. A manager who under-supervises tends to create feelings of isolation in staff, leading to staff ignoring the manager's directives. As a consequence, work may not be getting done and the manager can be regularly surprised by employees' actions/behaviours. Indeed this type of manager learns more about their staff from others outside the department or practice.

Second, consideration should be given to consulting, in confidence, with the person's colleagues and other managers if necessary. They may be privy to knowledge that may be helpful in dealing with the problem.

There are a number of factors to take into account when looking at possible causes of poor performance. They are set out in full in Box 7.7. In summary, they relate to the job description, adequate and appropriate training, the use of probationary periods, the quality and nature of personnel management in the practice, as well as the employee themselves.

Once the problem has been identified it needs to be analysed so that an action plan, which addresses the real causes of the poor work, can be devised. For example, it is little use arranging training if the real cause of poor work is personal problems at home or a destructive attitude towards work.

In discussions with the individual, managers should focus on the facts and examples of work (both good and bad) and ensure that the person is clear as to the standards required and the practice's expectations in reaching those standards. It is important for the short- and longer-term management of this sort of issue that records are kept of these discussions and that the individual receives, in writing, confirmation of the standard of

Box 7.7: Possible causes of poor performance

Job description
- too vague so the employee is not clear about the expectations of the job
- no job description
- out-of-date job description
- other staff are unaware of the job description; this is particularly common when staff change jobs and responsibilities

Training
- inadequate job induction training
- time is too limited
- planned without consulting the new member of staff or current staff
- training needs are not systematically identified
- expectations of performance are not articulated
- badly planned and haphazard
- new staff are made to feel they are intruding on the manager's time when asking for help
- the training requirements of new work are ignored or insufficiently addressed

Probationary periods
- lip service only is paid to the probationary period – someone has to be totally inadequate before their probationary period is extended
- discussion of performance is left until the probationary period is about to expire

Supervision and support
- over-supervising/under-supervising
- failure to discuss standards of work and how these will be monitored
- standards of performance are only addressed when things go wrong
- discussions are in the form of 'here's what is going wrong and this is how to do it'
- staff feel that errors are seen as failures rather than opportunities to learn
- emphasising quality while pushing for quantity

Personnel management
- inconsistent management of staff and between staff
- allowing conflict between staff to go unresolved

- lack of clear promotion criteria
- lack of clarity of roles and limits of authority
- delegating responsibility without the authority and/or the resources to do the work
- undermining the employee's self-confidence
- taking back delegated work
- changing job descriptions without consultation
- hovering and checking all work
- sarcastic comments
- bullying
- failing to model the standards expected by staff
- lack of cabinet responsibility amongst the management team
- applying the disciplinary procedure too soon
- not treating more mature employees with respect
- closing communication channels

The employee
- poorly matched to the requirements of the job and lacking the skills or potential to achieve results
- personal problems
- generally poor motivation and expectations of the organisation which cannot be fulfilled

work expected and that they are aware that their work is being monitored.

What often happens is that after a discussion there is a temporary improvement, which lulls the manager into thinking the problem has been resolved. As a result, the monitoring stops and review dates lapse. When the problem later resurfaces the manager has to start the procedure again from the beginning, as Example 7.4 illustrates.

Example 7.4

A part-time clerk in a busy practice produced slipshod work, which the practice manager thought was due to sheer carelessness resulting from the clerk's casual attitude to work. The manager took trouble to collect examples of her poor work and took her to one side. She made explicit the standards she required from the clerk and warned her that if there was not an improvement in her work, then a more formal meeting would be held. She arranged a further meeting in three week's time to discuss her review of the clerk's work. Nothing was put in writing.

The meeting was a real surprise to the clerk. No one had ever said anything before about her work. She immediately improved her standard of work. The manager was delighted and saw no reason to continue reviewing the clerk's work and the review meeting never took place. Some four months later, the manager realised that the clerk had slipped back to her old ways. However, as she had failed to closely monitor the work in the intervening period with appropriate warnings, she had to return to the first stage of an informal meeting and start the process again.

Most cases of poor performance, however, are resolved either through a sustained improvement in the work or by the individual deciding to look elsewhere for another job. However, if, after following the agreed action plan and providing the employee with the necessary support (training, coaching, time, equipment, etc.), the poor performance persists then the practice needs to consider issuing formal warnings and eventual dismissal. Chapter 8 details such dismissals. In these circumstances, following the procedure described, including keeping accurate records of all pertinent discussions and actions taken, is important for any dismissal to be fair.

8
Ending the contract of employment: conduct and capability issues

Chapters 4, 6 and 7 have discussed management problems that might result in the dismissal of an employee. These chapters have made clear that throughout the process of resolving an issue with an employee's conduct, ill health or competence, the manager needs to bear in mind that dismissal might be a possible outcome. These final two chapters therefore look at the legal context within which an employee's contract of employment can be terminated. Chapter 9 addresses the area of ending a contract of employment through redundancy, statutory bar or for some other substantial reason. This chapter addresses the reasons of conduct, capability and qualifications, defining each in turn and describing the most appropriate ways to approach each type of dismissal.

When the contract is ended by the employee, it is called resignation. When it is ended by the employer it is called dismissal. There are five fair reasons for dismissal.

The five fair reasons for dismissal

Section 98 of The Employment Rights Act 1996 recognises a number of potentially fair reasons for dismissal:

- conduct: misconduct and gross misconduct
- capability: qualifications, performance, ill health
- redundancy
- statutory bar
- some other substantial reason: business reorganisation, difficult working relationship, transfer of a business.

Fairness when dismissing an employee

The dismissal of a member of staff has legal implications and it is crucial that the reason for any such dismissal is fair and that the procedure used to dismiss is also fair. Staff with one year's service now have the right to claim unfair dismissal at an employment tribunal or through the ACAS Unfair Dismissal Procedure (see Chapter 9). To defend such action successfully, an employer must first prove that the employee has been dismissed for one of the five potentially fair reasons described above. He or she must then be able to demonstrate that, in all the circumstances, he or she acted fairly and properly in treating the reason as sufficient to dismiss the employee. This latter point is what is called the 'reasonableness test' and is discussed below.

Dismissing for reasons of conduct

Confronting personal and sensitive issues can be difficult for GPs (Irvine and Haman 2001). Historically, they have been reluctant to address disciplinary problems. Issuing a warning and dismissing staff are seen as actions which conflict with the profession's caring image. In addition, many employers feel constrained by the complexity of employment law and — wrongly — believe that dismissing an employee is almost impossible without risking employment tribunal proceedings. While it is undeniable that our conduct in work is affected by the rights and obligations imposed by law, employment regulations and particularly codes of practice are designed to foster, not hinder, good relations between employers and employees. Far from preventing employers taking disciplinary action, the law provides the framework within which disciplinary problems can be addressed.

The art is to use it properly and fairly, bearing in mind that most employment law relating to terminating contracts of employment embodies what is good management practice. The ACAS Code of Practice on discipline (ACAS 2000) provides specific guidelines on the design and implementation of disciplinary rules and procedures.

Whether an employee is guilty of misconduct or not must be decided on the 'balance of probabilities'. An employer must show a tribunal that, in coming to a decision on the question of guilt, they have satisfied the test that the employer:

- had a genuine belief in the employee's guilt
- that belief was based on reasonable grounds following as much investigation into the case as was reasonable in the circumstances.

The degree of seriousness of the misconduct is an important factor in determining whether the employer has sufficient reason to dismiss.

Misconduct need not amount to gross misconduct to warrant dismissal. A less serious act of misconduct may justify dismissal when taken as the final stage of a disciplinary procedure under which previous warnings have been given. In these cases, the tribunal must consider whether it was 'within the range of reasonable responses for the employer to dismiss the employee in the circumstances' (Employment Rights Act 1996).

Tribunals will scrutinise an organisation's rules on discipline and dismissal and will expect the rules to set out examples of those offences which are considered acts of misconduct resulting in warnings being given to employees, and those offences which constitute gross misconduct and warrant summary dismissal for the first offence. Appendix F sets out the main principles of the ACAS Code of Practice on Disciplinary and Grievance Procedures in Employment. Internal disciplinary procedures should follow this Code.

Even when the rules are clear and consistently applied, the employer's assessment of the actual offence must be reasonable, i.e. a dismissal will not automatically be fair just because the rules say the offence will result in dismissal as Example 8.1 shows.

Example 8.1

The disciplinary rules in a large, busy practice stated that a breach of patient confidentiality was a dismissable offence. Trudy Single, a member of staff new to reception, was tricked by a newspaper journalist into revealing that a local person, who had recently been charged with a serious criminal offence, was a patient of the practice. She thus breached the disciplinary rules.

During the consequent disciplinary investigation it emerged that Trudy had no knowledge of the patient's impending court case and, more importantly, had not received training on telephone confidentiality or the procedure to be used if there was any doubt as to the identity of a caller. Given these facts the partners decided that, although the breach of confidentiality was serious, it would be unreasonable in all the circumstances to dismiss Trudy.

There are four key stages of dealing with a serious disciplinary issue:

1 investigation
2 disciplinary hearing
3 disciplinary decision
4 appeal.

Stage 1: the investigation

The first thing to remember when dealing with a disciplinary issue is that no matter how straightforward and clear-cut the disciplinary offence appears to be, a thorough investigation is necessary both to ensure fair play and to abide by the law. The investigation must ensure that the charge or allegations made against the employee are clear and that they are thoroughly investigated and recorded. The investigation should be conducted by a senior manager/partner who has not been implicated – either directly or indirectly – in the alleged disciplinary offence. An example of an investigation for persistent poor time keeping is given in Example 8.2

Example 8.2

Jill was a receptionist in the Anytown Practice and she had a poor history of time keeping. She had received several verbal warnings before disciplinary proceedings were instituted. The staff partner, Jeremy, carried out a thorough investigation and looked at:

- Jill's time-keeping record
- the record of warnings and the explanations Jill had given
- the review periods to ensure that they had been initiated and monitored
- the way other staff had been treated on this issue
- the practice's rules on punctuality.

As a result of this investigation Jeremy was satisfied that more formal disciplinary action needed to be taken.

An investigation of a serious first offence, such as theft, may also involve interviewing witnesses and testing out the allegations so that the employee is not asked to attend a disciplinary hearing for unsubstantiated or flimsy allegations.

If, after this exercise, it is clear that some form of action needs to be taken, the employee is informed. Here the ACAS Code is helpful. It contains recommendations for disciplinary procedures which must be regarded as golden rules:

- provide for workers to be informed of the complaints against them and where possible all relevant evidence before any hearing
- provide workers with an opportunity to state their case before any decisions are reached
- when deciding whether a disciplinary penalty is appropriate and what form it should take, it is important to bear in mind the need to act reasonably in all the circumstances.

Stage 2: the disciplinary hearing

Before the hearing

To ensure that the employee is able to defend himself or herself the available evidence needs to be given to him or her prior to the hearing. The purpose of the hearing is not to 'trip up' the employee, but to provide him or her with the opportunity to defend himself or herself, including any mitigating circumstances, so that the hearing comes to an informed and reasonable decision. It is important therefore that the employee is given sufficient time (at least two or three days) to prepare for the interview. The employee should also be encouraged to be accompanied by a colleague of their choice or, if a member of a trade union, then their trade union representative needs to be present. Chapter 5 details the role of the representative in disciplinary hearings.

At all times, and no matter how serious the complaint, an employee in this situation needs to be treated with respect and fairness. All disciplinary interviews, from issuing a verbal warning to dismissal, should be characterised by reasonableness and respect. Treating the employee like a naughty child and patronising attitudes will not foster good relations. Other staff will be keeping a close watch on the manner in which the problem is handled. Disciplinary issues which are managed hastily, inconsistently and with a loss of self-respect to the employee will lower staff morale in the practice.

Many employers have lost cases of unfair dismissal not because the reason was not valid but because they failed to follow the ACAS Code of Practice in their handling of the issue. Box 8.1 is a checklist for best practice in preparing for a disciplinary hearing.

Box 8.1: Pre-hearing check list

- do you know *exactly* what the complaint is?
- have you interviewed all relevant people and obtained all the data – dates, times, written statements, etc.?
- are you familiar with all this evidence and do you have it to hand?
- have you anticipated likely explanations which may be offered?
- have you to hand aides-mémoire of the main issues to be raised?
- are there sufficient copies available of any previous warnings relevant to the case?
- is the hearing panel briefed, have witnesses been contacted and will someone be taking notes?

The hearing

Disciplinary interviews can take the form of either informal discussions or formal hearings, depending on the seriousness of the disciplinary charge. It is the interview few people anticipate without some degree of anxiety. If the charge is serious and may lead to dismissal, the decision to deprive a person of their livelihood is not an easy one to take. At the least, claims of unfair dismissal will often succeed or fail on the employer's conduct prior to and during the disciplinary interview.

Often, the interview will not be the last stage in the procedure but a means of gaining an improvement in the employee. It should therefore be viewed constructively and thorough preparation is vital if a fair outcome, based on the facts, is to be achieved. Such preparation, including a thorough investigation, all helps in the management of the hearing.

If the disciplinary charge is not serious, the interview can be informal and can be the opportunity to counsel staff in improvements to conduct or performance. An apparently trivial matter may be indicative of more serious underlying problems; personal problems often manifest themselves at work in a deterioration in conduct or relations with colleagues. Example 8.3 illustrates this point.

Example 8.3

Jane was a long-standing receptionist in the Stanley Town practice. Her normal, polite behaviour changed over time and the practice manager received a number of complaints from patients about Jane's rather abrupt behaviour. During the informal meetings, the practice manager, Betty, had conducted with Jane to address the issue, she was unable to find any reason for Jane's behaviour. Eventually, after another complaint from a patient, she informed Jane that the formal disciplinary procedure was being invoked and that Jane would receive a letter giving her the details of the disciplinary hearing.

Before the hearing took place, Jane went to see Betty and confided in her that her eldest son Gary was in trouble with the police and had started taking heroin. Jane and her husband were extremely worried, if not traumatised, by these events and very embarrassed. She was feeling very stressed, hence her changed behaviour.

Betty decided that a disciplinary hearing would serve no purpose other than to increase Jane's anxiety and cause her to go off work sick. To support Jane, it was decided to move her to a vacant temporary clerical post, which was less pressurised and where she had no contact with the public. Her reception duties were covered by a temporary receptionist. It was agreed that the situation would be reviewed in two months' time when the clerical work to which she had been assigned would be coming to an end.

As with all interviews, ensure that it will be free of interruptions. If the hearing is likely to cause stress, arrange the time for late afternoon, allowing the employee to go straight home.

The practice's disciplinary procedures should indicate who should attend a disciplinary hearing. The following guidelines embody good practice:

- if possible, and particularly if the charge is serious, more than one manager should be in attendance. The ideal would be for one partner to chair, one partner or the practice manager to present the facts and another to take notes
- if the charge involves evidence from witnesses, these people should be in attendance. They should not, however, sit in on the whole interview as this would be inappropriate, comprising issues of confidentiality. If a crucial witness is not able or willing to attend, a signed statement should be available and should be sent to the employee prior to the hearing
- the partner responsible for hearing any appeal should not be in attendance. It is impossible to show that the principles of natural justice have been met if an appeal is heard by a partner who has participated in the disciplinary hearing.

However well-prepared, certain ground rules need to be observed in the conduct of a disciplinary hearing. Above all, the person conducting the hearing should maintain an open mind. The purpose is to ensure that all relevant facts and explanations are heard in order to establish whether disciplinary action is appropriate and, if so, the form it should take. It is not an interrogation nor an opportunity for employers to vent their anger or displeasure at the employee. The hearing itself should follow a fair and systematic sequence as set out in Box 8.2.

Box 8.2: Disciplinary hearing structure

The most satisfactory sequence is:

1 the person chairing explains:
- the purpose of the hearing
- how the hearing will be conducted
- who is and who will be present and why

2 the complaint(s) against the employee is then clearly explained and the facts revealed by the investigation are detailed. If witnesses are to give evidence they are then to be called in turn, leaving when each has finished

3 the employee is then invited to respond and allowed to question the witnesses

4 any response to or further questioning arising from points raised by the employee should wait until the employee has been given a fair hearing without interruption. The employee should also be given the right to call witnesses who may then be questioned by the panel

5 further discussions and questioning may be needed before all the facts are established. This discussion needs to be handled skilfully if it is not to degenerate into an unconstructive argument

6 if new evidence is revealed during the course of the hearing, further investigation may be needed. In these circumstances, do not be tempted or feel pressurised into reaching a decision without first suspending the hearing and investigating the new evidence. Once this second investigation has been completed the hearing can be reconvened

7 at the end of the hearing, the person chairing summarises the main points raised by both sides and the evidence which will be considered before reaching a decision. This summing up clarifies the issues under scrutiny and emphasises the fair and objective nature of the decision-making process.

Points 6 and 7 above are important to the overt demonstration that fairness, objectivity and justice are being applied to the case. One of the more common reasons why people sue for unfair dismissal is a grievance that they did not receive a fair hearing. Therefore being seen to be fair is as important as actually being fair.

As said earlier, disciplinary hearings are inevitably stressful events for all concerned, but particularly for the employee. It is not uncommon for the employee to become distressed or argumentative, but threatening behaviour or abusive language should not be tolerated. This type of extreme behaviour should be treated as misconduct and the hearing adjourned until a later date when both the issue in hand and the subsequent mis-conduct can be dealt with together.

A major difficulty arises when an employee refuses to respond during the hearing. It is important to establish the reason why the employee is refusing to participate. If it involves a personal problem, offer the employee the opportunity to discuss the matter with the most appropriate partner or the practice manager. If this offer is rejected or if the refusal to respond does not involve a personal issue, the employee should be advised that such a refusal will mean that the panel cannot take into account any mitigating circumstances.

Stage 3: the decision

Once all the evidence has been heard, the hearing should then be adjourned before reconvening and announcing a decision. There should be no pressure to reach a decision quickly. Depending on the complexity and seriousness of the case, a day or two may be needed to make a decision. The time taken, however, should not be so long as to cause undue stress to the employee.

Even in the most straightforward cases, the practice of adjourning – even if only for 10 minutes – before making a decision is strongly recommended. It demonstrates that careful consideration is being given and it allows time to consider the type of disciplinary action to be taken, which must follow the organisation's own disciplinary procedure.

Once a decision has been reached, the hearing is reconvened and the employee told of the decision. If the decision involves disciplinary action short of dismissal, do:

- specify the improvements that you require to be made
- inform the employee of any help the practice can offer, e.g. further training
- specify when you expect the improvements to be made
- specify any review period

- specify any penalties that may be incurred for further breaches
- specify the lifespan of the warning
- explain the right to appeal and the procedure to be used.

With the exception of verbal warnings, all disciplinary hearings resulting in disciplinary action should be followed by a letter confirming:

- the reason(s) why the hearing was held
- who attended
- if the employee was not accompanied, it is advisable to include in the letter a statement to the effect that 'despite being aware of your right to be accompanied, you chose to attend the hearing alone'
- the disciplinary action taken and the consequences, if appropriate, of any further breaches of the disciplinary rules
- any improvements that are required, when they are to be made and any review period
- the right to appeal and the appeal procedure
- if the decision to dismiss has been reached, the notice period or pay in lieu of notice.

Box 8.3 is the disciplinary warning letter sent to Jill the receptionist from Anytown Practice.

Box 8.3: Disciplinary warning letter

Dear Jill,

I am writing to you to confirm the details of the disciplinary hearing you attended this morning with myself and Susan Right, practice manager. You exercised your right to be accompanied by a fellow employee, who was Ginny March.

As you are aware from my letter to you of ..... informing you of the hearing and detailing your time keeping over the last six months, the purpose of the hearing was to address your punctuality record.

During the course of the hearing you made the point that you were not a 'morning person' and that you had trouble getting up in the morning. Regrettably I cannot treat this as an acceptable explanation. I am therefore issuing you with a written warning that, unless there is an immediate and sustained improvement in your time-keeping record, then serious consideration will be given to issuing you with a final written warning.

This written warning follows two verbal warnings issued to you on ..... and ...... Your time keeping will continue to be closely monitored and Susan will formally review it every two weeks for the next three months. This warning will stay on your personnel file for one year.

You are aware of the extra burden your regular lateness places on your colleagues and I sincerely hope that you can improve this aspect of your work and that there will be no need to hold another disciplinary hearing.

You have the right to appeal against this decision. Should you wish to do so, a letter stating your reasons for appealing should be addressed to Dr Harry within five working days of receiving this letter.

Yours sincerely,

Dr Jeremy Inglenook

Stage 4: the appeal

The ACAS Code recommends that an employee be given the right to appeal. This right and the procedure should be clearly stated when the disciplinary decision is given and again in the disciplinary letter, as Box 8.3 above shows. The appeal is the employee's opportunity to either restate 'their side of the story' or to present new evidence in their favour.

The appeal should be to a partner who has not been involved in the original decision. He or she needs to become familiar with all the facts. If not satisfied with the thoroughness of the original investigation or the conduct of the disciplinary hearing, or if new evidence is presented by the employee, the partner will need to conduct a further investigation.

After careful consideration, the employee and the members of the disciplinary hearing should then be informed of the result of the employee's appeal. Informing the employee of this decision verbally and/or in writing will depend on the process described in the practice's appeal procedure.

The decision will be *either* to uphold the original decision *or* to overrule the original decision. If the decision is the latter, then any lesser disciplinary action should be specified, e.g. a decision to issue a written warning may be reduced to a verbal warning. Example 8.4 shows what happened when Jill appealed.

Example 8.4

Jill appealed against her written warning. In her letter to Dr Harry, she stated that other members of staff were also often late for work but had not received any warnings and this unfairness was her reason for appealing.

Dr Harry duly investigated the time keeping of other employees and how Susan Right, the practice manager, had dealt with staff who were late for work.

He discovered that Susan had designed and communicated clear rules on time keeping and all staff were aware that any person who was late more than three times in any four-week period was spoken to. Over the past year two members of staff had been counselled about their time keeping but as there had been no repetition of tardiness after the counselling interviews in either case, no further action had been taken.

Dr Harry therefore could not find any reason to alter the hearing's decision to issue a written warning and replied accordingly to Jill.

Hopefully, most practices will never need to institute disciplinary proceedings; most day-to-day problems are solved informally. However, it is impossible to predict or anticipate human behaviour accurately. It is far better for relations if disciplinary rules and procedures are firmly established before rather than after an event which may occasion disciplinary action. The very fact that there are no established rules and procedures may make any subsequent dismissal unfair.

It is also only good management practice, regardless of the statutory requirements, to ensure that all staff, regardless of length of service, are treated fairly and are fully aware of the rules relating to work and the penalties for breaching those rules. Above all they need to be aware of the procedure for handling any such breaches.

The partners and practice manager may feel uncomfortable in establishing written rules and procedures and consequently adopting a more formal and detached approach when handling a disciplinary issue. However, such an approach is essential to the effective performance of the practice and in the prevention of tribunal proceedings. Indeed, the staff of today expect and want clear rules and procedures in this area of workplace relations; they give security to employees that any allegations against them of misconduct will be treated in a professional and considered way, following the laws of natural justice.

Dismissing for reasons of capability

Capability is defined in Section 98(3)(a) of The Employment Rights Act as being assessed by reference to skill, aptitude, health or any other physical or mental quality. The two most common causes justifying dismissals on grounds of capability, or rather lack of it, are dismissals of employees who are regarded as simply incompetent and dismissals relating to ill health that has led to prolonged or frequent absences from work. This section on capability therefore deals first with performance, then ill health and finally a third category, that of qualifications. These are defined as meaning any degree, diploma or other academic, technical or professional qualification relevant to the position the employee held.

Performance

Where an employee is dismissed for incapacity or incompetence, tribunals, as with judgements on dismissals for misconduct, pose the 'honest belief' question – is there an honest belief, by the employer, that the employee was incapable or incompetent? Clearly, it is important therefore that again, as with misconduct dismissals, no dismissal is considered without first undertaking a thorough investigation.

Providing evidence of poor performance

First and foremost the employer must be able to demonstrate, at the time of the dismissal, the existence of a reasonable belief that the employee's performance was incompetent, incapable or otherwise flawed. The employer must show that there were reasonable grounds for concluding that the employee was not capable of performing as required. Evidence needs to be gathered and substantiated. There may be measurable evidence, for example productivity data, quality inspection and control measures, targets and so on. There may be complaints about the employee's work from patients, clients, other staff, supervisors or managers. The inability to meet agreed targets or to perform in accordance with individual objectives set can underpin the employer's loss of confidence in an employee's performance. Even a single or isolated act of incompetence could provide necessary evidence.

The importance of employers recording and documenting an employee's poor performance cannot be overstated. Failure to do this can result in the employer being unable to establish that poor performance was a reason for dismissal. There is also the possibility that a tribunal might be led to the conclusion that incompetence or incapability was not the real reason for the dismissal. It is important therefore that all documentary evidence supports the assertion of incompetence. A positive appraisal, a performance-related bonus payment or a glowing reference can all undermine the employer's case.

Chapter 7 details the different approaches of improving an employee's performance. This chapter now looks at how such approaches should fit into a fair procedure for handling a dismissal and how to effect such a dismissal.

Following a fair procedure

If a performance-related dismissal is to be fair, it should include the elements set out in Box 8.4.

Box 8.4: Elements of a fair dismissal for poor performance

- investigation or appraisal of the employee's performance
- account taken of any factors affecting performance, e.g. personal problems, inadequate resources or poor training
- clear communication to the employee as to why or how his or her performance is unsatisfactory
- discussion with the employee about the poor performance and its causes – these discussions might reveal a personal or health problem, or personality clash with another colleague, which in turn might suggest some alternative method of dealing with the problem
- advice or direction to the employee as to how his or her performance should be improved
- sufficient warnings that the consequence of continued poor performance will be a final warning or dismissal
- a reasonable time period allowed within which the employee is to improve performance or to demonstrate competence
- monitoring of the employee's progress during this time
- sufficient support, supervision and, where necessary, training or retraining so as to allow the employee to reach the required performance standards
- where appropriate, consideration of moving the employee to alternative employment. This would be appropriate where poor performance is due to a person being over-promoted or transferred to work for which he or she is not suited
- issuing a final warning, in writing, before the final decision to dismiss is made

In addition to following one's own practice guidelines and procedures on handling poor performance, the above elements also need to be observed. In the absence of a specific internal procedure, the practice's own disciplinary procedure can provide a guide as to how to handle the formal meetings with an employee. Whatever the procedure, the employee should always be given a fair hearing and an opportunity to state his or her case or to contribute to the resolution of the problem.

Experience shows that employees at tribunals have very selective memories and without the minutes of meetings and copies of letters, it is common to hear that interviews never took place, nor were warnings received. All such hearings and discussions therefore should be minuted and decisions confirmed in writing.

When dealing with a senior employee or professionally qualified member of staff, it may not be necessary to spell out the consequences of continued poor performance as Example 8.5 illustrates.

Example 8.5

The senior partner of the William Street Surgery was informed by the practice's accountant that the practice's insurance premiums on equipment and premises had not been paid for the past six months. The partners were appalled and immediately instructed the practice manager, Jerry Ranking, to resume and back-date the payments. No formal warning was given, but they made it clear to Jerry that they were angry and concerned about this lapse in his performance.

One month later the practice fell victim to vandalism and theft and in one night suffered the loss of four computers and one video camera. The reception area was also badly vandalised, necessitating complete redecoration and refurbishment.

When a claim was submitted, the practice was informed by the insurance company that, despite several reminders, the practice manager had failed to renew the insurance; they had assumed that the practice had changed to another insurance company. This was not the case and the practice was left with a hefty bill.

Although Jerry had not been formally warned that his omission to insure the practice was a possible dismissable issue, the partners were advised by an employment law expert that a dismissal on grounds of capability would be fair, as insuring the practice was clearly Jerry's responsibility and, given his senior position and the seriousness of the repeated failure to undertake this responsibility, Jerry could expect to be dismissed.

If the employer has provided adequate training and support, supervision and resources, it may not be reasonable to expect the employer to invest further in the employee short of giving him or her a final chance to correct the problem. The size of the organisation will also be relevant, both in terms of how long an opportunity is given to improve and whether alternative employment should be considered.

The nature and character of the employee is also relevant. For example, a long-serving employee may be given more leeway than an employee with shorter service or a probationer.

Ill health

Chapter 7 details the different ways a practice can manage absence effectively and the steps to take when approaching a potential or actual long-term ill health problem of a member of staff. This section now looks at the procedure to adopt when the practice eventually decides that the employee can no longer continue being employed.

To ensure a fair process, employers need to show that the ill health adversely affected the employee's performance or ability to undertake his or her work. It is also important for employers to demonstrate that even if the employee could not do their current work, there was no other type of work available for which they would have been capable.

More commonly, dismissals through illness arise where an employer is not prepared to tolerate the effect of an employee's absence any longer. The absence places an additional burden on colleagues and, more particularly, staff morale may be damaged by such absence and the employer's tolerance of it. In these cases, the basic questions which have to be determined are first, whether under the circumstances the employer can be expected to wait any longer for the employee to return to good health and return to work. And second, if so, how much longer can the employer wait, keeping the employee's job open?

Following a fair procedure

First, tribunals will expect an employer to establish that there was a need to have the work done. It is usually a fairly straightforward task to meet this expectation.

Second, a full investigation of the case needs to be undertaken. Chapter 7 details the process of obtaining medical evidence. Once such a report is received it should be investigated and not necessarily accepted at face value, otherwise the employer may have difficulties establishing the thoroughness of any investigation. For example, a medical report states that an employee is suffering from agoraphobia which is treatable and yet the employer has first-hand evidence that the employee in question is regularly seen out and about the locality. In this scenario, before accepting the medical report at face value, the investigation would include meeting with the employee and discussing the contradictory evidence.

If more than one medical report is available, they may conflict. Where conflicting medical reports are received, unless there is an option to receive a third medical report, the practice will be justified in relying on its own medical adviser, who should not be a partner of the practice. Equally, an employee can refuse to submit to a medical examination. Where this occurs, the practice should write to the employee that, without such a report, the practice will have to take a decision based only on the evidence already available to it.

Decisions to dismiss usually take place once the employee is nearing or at the end of their sick-pay entitlement. Indeed, it could be difficult to demonstrate fairness if an employee is dismissed before taking all of his or her sick-pay entitlement. This does not mean that discussions about termination should wait until the sick pay has expired.

Once the decision has been taken to dismiss, the impending termination of employment will be easier to raise and discuss if regular visiting (see Chapter 7) has been part of the practice's relationship with the ill employee than if the employee has been managed at arm's length. Part of these discussions will involve the payments due to the employee and the contract of employment will determine the minimum due. Discussions will also include notice period – regardless of the fact that the employee cannot work, he or she is entitled to notice with pay. If the practice decides to dismiss before the sick pay has expired, then these discussions should include 'rolling up' the employee's remaining sick-pay entitlement as part of the termination payment. Example 8.6 illustrates this point.

Example 8.6

Natasha, a young receptionist, fell ill with depression and took long-term sick leave. Penny, the practice's manager, kept in regular contact with her and after three months, when Natasha's condition appeared to be deteriorating rather than improving, she sought and received Natasha's permission to obtain a medical report from her consultant.

The report stated that Natasha's condition was serious and that there was little possibility of her returning to work in the foreseeable future.

Given this prognosis, Penny and Natasha discussed the possibility of Natasha leaving the practice. Natasha was relieved, as she had been feeling guilty that her job had been kept open when she herself

> could see that it would be a very long time before she could return to any type of work.
>
> Natasha's dismissal was processed and in addition to receiving a month's notice, with pay, she also received the remainder of her sick-pay entitlement, which amounted to three months' salary at half pay. By doing this, and with the medical report as crucial evidence if later challenged, the practice had fulfilled its contractual obligations to Natasha.

Ill health dismissals and disability

One of the major pieces of legislation which has had a profound effect on ill health dismissals has been the Disability Discrimination Act. Chapter 3 details this Act. It is particularly pertinent when deciding to dismiss an employee on grounds of ill health.

If an employee who is on long-term sick leave comes under the definition of disability, then the employer must consider further ways of avoiding dismissal before any final decision is made to terminate employment. These further ways involve looking at making reasonable adjustments if that would prevent the dismissal of the employee. Such adjustments include altering the physical features of the premises and/or modifying working arrangements. This latter modification may include reallocation of duties, transferring to another job, altering hours of work, starting and finishing times, relocation, installing specialist equipment, working from home, etc. Clearly, for most practices some of these adjustments would be unreasonable and tribunals will take into consideration the cost-benefit ratio of the possible adjustment, size of the organisation and resources available, and also how much information the employer gathered before making the decision on an adjustment. This information gathering includes whether or not the employer contacted disability groups, who are a valuable source of information and may have solutions to what may appear insurmountable problems.

Qualifications

Dismissals due to lack of qualifications are rare because it will be apparent to an employer on first employing someone that the person does not have the necessary qualifications to satisfactorily and/or lawfully discharge his or her employment. The most common example of where a qualification fundamental to the job is the reason for dismissal is the loss of a driving licence, as illustrated in Example 8.7

Example 8.7

Adam Burns was the practice manager of Hill Street Practice, which operated from two sites of similar sizes. As a rural practice there was no public transport between the two sites, and a car was the only way of getting from one site to the other. A driving licence was therefore essential for the practice manager, as he had to manage both sites and needed to visit each at least three times a week.

After two years in the post, Adam was found guilty of dangerous driving and lost his licence for three years. This meant that he was unable to do his job and it was not practicable to get someone else to chauffeur him. Also there was no local taxi service. Given all these factors, and the absence of any alternative employment that the practice could offer him, they regrettably dismissed him on grounds of qualifications.

As Example 8.7 illustrates, before dismissing, employers need to consider if there are any alternative ways in which the person can do their job without personally driving a vehicle or if there is any alternative employment to which the employee can be transferred.

In conclusion, it is clearly in the interests of good management practice and staff relations for practices to develop their own disciplinary and performance procedures, following the appropriate codes of practice, and very important for them to ensure that they are applied consistently and fairly, acting reasonably at all times.

9
Ending the contract of employment: redundancy, statutory bar or some other substantial reason

This chapter addresses the three other fair reasons for dismissal: redundancy, statutory bar and some other substantial reason. The last two reasons are rarely used and therefore this chapter is primarily concerned with redundancy. This chapter (and book) ends with an outline of the new ACAS Arbitration Scheme, which will be of interest to smaller organisations who wish to avoid the lengthy and costly business of employment tribunals.

Redundancy

The issue of redundancy and/or redeployment is a very uncomfortable one but it is an inescapable fact of modern life. The handling of a redundancy is prescribed in statute, in particular The Employment Rights Act 1996, and current case law. In addition to observing the law, any employer considering declaring an employee redundant also needs to be aware of, and sensitive to, the emotions surrounding a redundancy in the workplace.

What this means is that the practice needs to think through very carefully not only the legalities of the process, but also the emotional and practical needs of the employee, the effects on the staff who are staying and the people in the practice who are actually handling the redundancy. A hasty, ill-considered approach can result in a level of uncertainty among staff, which can adversely affect morale and performance. In all the issues described below, reference is made to the value of looking beyond the legal requirements at each stage.

The legal background

On the subject of redundancy, The Employment Rights Act 1996 states that:

an employee who is dismissed shall be taken to be dismissed by reason of redundancy if the dismissal is attributable wholly or mainly to:

the fact that his employer has ceased, or intends to cease, to carry on the business for the purposes of which the employee was employed by him, or has ceased, or intends to cease, to carry on that business in the place where the employee was so employed,

or

the fact that the requirements of that business for employees to carry out work of a particular kind in the place where he was so employed, have ceased or diminished or are expected to cease or diminish.

In other words, when the work or type of work undertaken by employees has ceased or diminished, a redundancy may occur. This can include transferring work to another location or altering the type of work undertaken in the organisation.

It is not unusual for employers to try to use the label of redundancy to dismiss staff they no longer wish to employ because they are not satisfied or happy with their performance or conduct at work. Tribunals are very aware of this practice and scrutinise such claims of unfair dismissal thoroughly.

The issues to consider

There are a number of key elements to consider when proposing to dismiss an employee on grounds of redundancy as set out in Box 9.1.

Box 9.1: Key elements of a redundancy

- consultation
- objective criteria for selection
- redundancy payments
- notice periods
- alternative work
- trial periods
- time off with pay

Consultation

The Employment Rights Act 1996 places an obligation on employers to consult recognised trade unions at the earliest opportunity. This means as soon as the employer proposes to dismiss employees. Although few practices deal with and/or have recognised agreements with trade unions, a House of Lords ruling in *Polkey v AV Dayton Services Ltd* (1987) IRLR 503 is relevant. This ruling stated that employers must consult individuals who may be dismissed. It is interpreted as meaning that, even where there is no recognised trade union, employers must consult those individuals they propose to declare redundant.

The purpose of the consultation is to inform employees of what the employer proposes and to listen to the employee's views on how to avoid or mitigate the effects of redundancy. Consequently, it is advisable to offer a period of consultation of no less than two weeks during which time these consultative discussions take place. It is only after this consultation period has expired that any redundancy notices should be issued.

It is important to note that even if the reasons for redundancy are completely fair, a tribunal may still judge the dismissal to be unfair on procedural grounds, including lack of consultation. Such consultation should include putting the proposal in writing, giving the information outlined in Box 9.2.

Box 9.2: Consultation information

- the reasons for the proposals
- the number and descriptions of employees it is proposed to dismiss as redundant
- the total number of employees of that description employed in the establishment
- the proposed method of selecting the employees who may be dismissed
- the proposed method of carrying out the dismissals including the period over which the dismissals will take effect

---

Case law has demonstrated that consultation must be meaningful and not a sham. The employer cannot go through the charade of listening to representations and then imposing a predetermined decision. This was made clear in the *TGWU v Ledbury Preserves (1982) Ltd (No 1)* (1985) IRLR 412, where the Employer Appeal Tribunal (EAT) said that:

> There must be sufficient meaningful consultation before notices of dismissal are sent out. The consultation must not be a show exercise; there must be time for union representatives who are consulted to consider properly the proposals that are being put to them.

Selection

The issues listed in Box 9.2 are not placed chronologically. Employers will often have some idea as to which employees are likely to be declared redundant before the consultation process begins. On the other hand, part of the consultation process can include discussions on the method and criteria used in selecting staff for redundancy. The selection process is probably the most important element in achieving a fair redundancy.

Where only one job is being made redundant and only one person undertakes that type of work, then selection is fairly straightforward – it is the person doing the job. Selection becomes problematic where a number of staff undertake similar work, some of which is no longer needed.

In selecting staff for redundancy, it is clearly vital to the smooth running of the practice that individuals with the key skills essential to its day-to-day running are retained. Accordingly, an objective process of evaluating employees' skills and suitability is important. This process of drawing up selection criteria appropriate to a practice's needs is now described.

The system of 'last in first out' (LIFO) to select redundant staff is no longer the only way of selecting for redundancy. More sophisticated criteria for selection are being used by many organisations in order to ensure that a balanced workforce is maintained, which can offer appropriate skill, flexibility and adaptability. Whatever the criteria used, the method of selection must be reasonable and objective and communicated to affected employees so that they are able to judge whether they themselves have been fairly selected. This is especially important where the functions that are no longer required are spread out among a number of different staff so that there is no easily made single decision.

Until the demise of fundholding, redundancies in general practice were rare, with few (if any) redundancy policies or procedures developed. However, if a practice decides that a redundancy situation is looming, it is good practice to develop a set of criteria that the practice can apply in selecting staff for redundancy. The earlier this is done the better. The selection criteria need to strike a balance between consistency and flexibility and it is helpful to bear in mind that a tribunal may well be in the position of scrutinising these criteria for fairness and objectivity.

Criteria should not reflect the personal opinions of individuals and should be verifiable by reference to data. Criteria which are often used (in no particular order) include:

- ability and performance: if these criteria are used there should be sustained written evidence of objective appraisal
- skills and experience: again evidence of an objective assessment would be necessary. A record of the types of jobs held by individuals, skills obtained, courses attended and qualifications gained are all acceptable sources of evidence to support the assessment of a person's skills and experience
- attendance: attendance records need to be accurate and up to date. The reasons for the absences must also be considered to ensure that they are not linked with disability or work-related illnesses such as stress. Maternity absences must be explicitly excluded otherwise this criterion will fall foul of the Sex Discrimination Act 1975. The period over which absences are considered should not be longer than is reasonable
- disciplinary record: again, the period over which this record is considered should not be longer than is reasonable
- length of service (LIFO): although this is probably the easiest to administer it may not address a practice's needs.

When drawing up selection criteria it is important to bear in mind the points listed in Box 9.3.

The dismissal of an employee selected for redundancy is likely to be found unfair if the employee was selected for one of the reasons listed in Box 9.4

Box 9.3: Points to remember when selecting criteria

- include factors which are capable of objective measurement
- avoid vague factors such as 'attitude', which allow for personal prejudices and are difficult to support with evidence
- be careful when assessing output, work rate or attendance records as they may be distorted by an individual's disability or time taken off work for trade union activity
- ensure assessments are made accurately and fairly; double check that any figures are accurate

Box 9.4: Unfair selection for redundancy

- the selection is in breach of a customary arrangement or agreed procedure, unless there are special reasons to justify the breach
- the selection is for membership and/or activities associated with a trade union, or non-membership, or refusing to become a member of a trade union
- the selection is discriminatory on grounds of race, sex, pregnancy, maternity, trade union membership or disability

Redundancy payments

Only those employees who have worked for the same employer for two years or more are legally entitled to a redundancy payment, although as stated in Chapter 5, employees with only one year's service have the right to claim unfair dismissal. When calculating payments, service before the age of 18 does not count. Employees who have reached the normal retirement age for their place of work, or are aged 65, are not eligible for statutory redundancy payment regardless of the number of years service or hours worked per week.

The Department of Education and Employment produces a booklet (DoEE 1990) with details of calculating redundancy payments. Statutory redundancy payment is determined by the employee's age, length of service and salary. When calculating a week's pay there is a statutory maximum limit, currently £230 per week. The maximum limit is now index-linked each year. A rough guide is given in Box 9.5

Box 9.5: A guide to redundancy payments

For each complete year of service, up to a maximum of 20 years, an employee is entitled to:

- half a week's pay for each year of service from age 18 and over but under 22
- one week's pay for each year of service from age 22 and over but under 41
- one and a half week's pay for each year of employment from age 41 and over but under retirement age

The redundancy payments described in Box 9.5 are the payments employers are bound in law to provide for eligible staff. Employers can of course offer enhanced severance payments and indeed such enhancements can do much to alleviate some of the distress experienced by all concerned when members of staff lose their jobs through redundancy.

Notice periods

As with any dismissal, redundant employees are entitled to their contractual notice period or pay in lieu of notice. It is for the employer to decide whether or not they wish the employee to work all, some or none of the notice period. The circumstances of the redundancy may be such that it would be better for both the redundant employee and the organisation if pay in lieu of notice is given. It also offers the leaver the opportunity to use the time to seek other employment. However, pay in lieu of notice should be used with care and sensitivity as Example 9.1 illustrates.

Example 9.1

When facing the demise of fundholding, the King Street Practice had to make their two fundholding clerks, Jeannie and Anna, redundant. The partners followed a fair and legal procedure leading up to the final meeting with the two staff to confirm the decision to dismiss and to give them their dismissal notices.

This final meeting was held with the senior partner at 5.00 pm where he confirmed that, with great regret, their jobs were being made redundant from today. In order to let them have time to look for other work, he advised them that they would have pay in lieu of notice and could leave the practice immediately after clearing their desks.

Although Jeannie and Anna had been fully consulted about the proposed redundancies and knew from previous meetings the reasons they had been selected, being asked to leave in this manner was extremely distressing. They felt as if they had been sacked for some wrongdoing, that being asked to leave immediately was some sort of punishment and implied a loss of trust in them, with no time to say goodbye or plan for their departure.

What, up until this point, had been an exemplary redundancy process, was now damaged and the rest of the staff viewed the partners as heartless and unfeeling and began to feel insecure themselves.

There are advantages to the employee in working their notice period. If the employer is willing, the employee can use the facilities of the practice, such as secretarial services for preparing CVs or using the telephone to contact future employers. There is no legal requirement to offer these services, but it makes good sense to offer whatever help is possible and appropriate to the circumstances of each case. Not only is the practice helping the redundant employee to get back into the job market, but it is also showing the rest of the staff that it is a considerate employer even when tough decisions have had to be made.

Alternative work

Even when the decision is made to declare a person's job redundant, the question of alternative employment is relevant to the reasonableness of the dismissal. A claim for unfair dismissal may arise if the employer has failed to undertake reasonable steps to offer employees alternative jobs within the organisation. Tribunals take into consideration the resources of the employer. A small general practice, for example, would not be expected to be able to offer alternative employment to the same degree (if at all) as a multinational organisation.

What constitutes suitable alternative employment is determined by a number of factors, including pay, status, location, hours of work and the working environment.

Practices are small organisations, however, and it will be clear early on in the process whether or not there is suitable work for the employee to do. In *Thomas & Betts Manufacturing Ltd v Harding* (1980) IRLR 255, the Court of Appeal ruled that an employer should do what they can *so far as is reasonable* to seek to provide alternative work.

Where alternative work is found within the organisation, the employee must be offered the new position before the notice period of the redundant post has expired. Where the new post is very similar to the redundant position in terms of the type of work and the terms and conditions of employment, any refusal by the employee to accept the offer could be viewed as unreasonable by the employer, and the employer could refuse to make a redundancy payment. Example 9.2 illustrates this point.

Example 9.2

The practice manager in a busy urban practice retired. Her successor examined the manpower needs of the practice. She came to the conclusion, which was supported by the partners, that there were too many nurse hours for the current and future requirements of the practice. The three full-time nurses were consulted and one of them, Sadie, volunteered for redundancy. However, before her notice period expired, one of her nurse colleagues died unexpectedly. The deceased worked mainly in health promotion, while Sadie's main responsibilities lay in the treatment room.

Sadie was duly advised that the vacancy resulting from the sudden death of her colleague would be offered to her as suitable alternative employment to the redundancy. As the job differed slightly from her current post, she would be entitled to a four-week trial period (see below).

Sadie refused this offer and insisted that the redundancy go ahead. The partners refused and told her that if she left the practice before trying out the job offered, they would be under no legal obligation to pay her a redundancy payment. Sadie reluctantly stayed with the practice but was disgruntled and her performance was not up to the expected standard. All were relieved when she resigned some four months later to join a private nursing agency.

Employers have to weigh up the advantages and pitfalls of exercising this right not to make a redundancy payment where an offer of suitable employment is refused. A situation can arise where the employee agrees reluctantly to accept the offer. Employing unwilling staff who are not working for the practice through choice can be more expensive in the long term than making a redundancy payment. As Example 9.2 illustrates, the disaffection felt by the member of staff can affect their performance at work and the morale of the surgery.

Trial period

Where a practice is able to offer alternative work to a member of staff under threat or notice of redundancy, the employee has the right to try it out. This period of trying out the new post is called the trial period, which should be for no less than four weeks, or longer if the employer agrees. This trial period enables the employee and the employer to decide whether the new job is suitable without the employee forfeiting the right to a redundancy payment.

Should the employee leave during the trial period because the new post is not suitable, or should the employer dismiss the employee due to their unsuitability, the employee leaves with a redundancy payment and is treated as if the redundancy took place at the expiration of the original notice period. However, if the employee is dismissed during the trial period for a reason unconnected with redundancy, for example gross misconduct, then he or she may lose the redundancy entitlement. In such a case, the employer may have to justify the dismissal in the normal way before a tribunal and all the usual disciplinary procedures should be applied.

Alternative offers of employment, and particularly those which attract a trial period, should be detailed in writing, stating the date when the trial period starts and finishes, and the measures which will be used to assess the employee's suitability. All offers of alternative work must be made before the employee's contractual notice period has expired and taken up either immediately after the end of the old job or after an interval of not more than four weeks.

Time off with pay

Employees with two years' service and who are under formal notice of redundancy have the right to reasonable time off with pay, in working hours, to look for work or to make arrangements for training for future employment. A tribunal can make a financial award against the employer if they unreasonably refuse this right to employees under notice of redundancy. However, it is good management practice, regardless of the years of service, to allow staff paid time off to make such plans for their future.

The personnel management of redundancy

If the practice handles a redundancy insensitively, it is remembered by those who stay as well as by those who are being made redundant. Trust and confidence can be more easily damaged by a badly handled redundancy than almost any other single event in an organisation. Once the process of consultation and selection has been undertaken, the communication of the decision should be given the highest priority in the management of the practice at that time.

The meeting where the proposal to select the person is communicated should be very short, as most people, when given news of this nature, cease to hear anything after the initial announcement. It may be necessary to arrange a second meeting where further details of the redundancy can be discussed.

While there are no precise statutory rules on how these individual consultations should be managed, best practice would involve the process described in Box 9.6.

Box 9.6: Individual consultations

- the employee should be encouraged to be accompanied by a colleague
- a full explanation should be given as to why the employee's particular job may be affected by redundancy and the details of the selection criteria
- individuals should be encouraged to discuss what is proposed and given time to express any concerns about their selection; the meeting may need to be adjourned to enable sufficient time for the employee to think through any concerns they may have
- all the factors relating to the proposed redundancy should be to hand so that the employee is in possession of as many facts as possible; these factors would include redundancy payments and whether pay in lieu of notice will be given to those finally selected
- any points made by the employee should be seriously considered and discussed including the possibility of any alternative work (if any)

- redundancy lists should be finalised only after the individual consultation process is complete
- a further meeting with the employee will need to be arranged, and again he or she should be accompanied by a colleague, to confirm the selection, issue notice of dismissal, and details of the support and help the practice is able to offer to staff

Even before redundancy notices have been issued and during the consultation process, employees may have feelings of anger and even bereavement which need to be explored and dealt with before a constructive attitude to opportunities for new work can be adopted. The practice should not be tempted to undertake this counselling role in-house. If a member of staff is experiencing these emotions, even if counselling is a specialty of the practice, the practice must retain the detached employer role. A reputable 'out-placement' company can do much to help redundant staff or, of course, the employee can be referred to a variety of professionals who can offer counselling.

The distress of redundancy cannot be overemphasised, and most people need reassurance in their worth as employees and practical help in seeking new employment. Frequently, the employee does not realise that the decision to dismiss was difficult and that it does not reflect on their value as a person. Reassurance needs to be made verbally explicit and sincere expressions of regret should be included in the letter of termination of employment. Providing open references, contacting other practices that may have vacancies, and providing resources and assistance to the employee will help alleviate some of the more immediate stresses on the individual and on the practice. The staff and colleagues who remain may go through a period of guilt and grieving, unsure of their own futures in the practice. They too need to be given reassurance. Handling a redundancy professionally, sympathetically and generously (both in money and the time) can do much to maintain the morale of the staff and the partners of the practice.

Statutory bar

Dismissal for the reason of statutory bar is when an employee loses a legal authority or licence to carry out the work for which they are employed. The medical profession offers the classic examples under this category of doctors being suspended or struck off the GMC register, and nurses losing their licence with the United Kingdom Consultative Committee.

As with all other types of dismissal, an appropriate investigation needs to be undertaken substantiating the evidence of the statutory bar and with all other circumstances being taken into account before deciding to dismiss the employee.

Some other substantial reason

The category of 'some other substantial reason' (SOSR) is designed to be a catch-all, and to cover circumstances not covered by the reasons specified in Section 98 of The Employment Rights Act 1996. Therefore it covers any reason for dismissing an employee, provided that the reason is a substantial one and not a whim of the employer. Examples of some other substantial reasons are set out in Box 9.7.

Box 9.7: Examples of some other substantial reasons

- **a necessary business reorganisation:** where consequent dismissals do not fall within the legal definition of redundancy
- **transfer of a business:** this comes within the meaning of the Transfer Undertakings (Protection of Employment) Regulations 1981
- **breakdown of trust and confidence:** where the actions or omissions on the part of the employee leads to the breakdown and where it cannot be categorised as misconduct or gross misconduct
- **personality differences:** if difficulties in the working relationships between staff escalate and detrimentally affect the business of an organisation

Tribunals approach dismissals on the grounds of SOSR with caution. They are particularly sensitive to employers using SOSR as an excuse to dismiss a member of staff whose actions cannot be contrived to fit into one of the other four categories of dismissal (conduct and capability described in Chapter 8, and redundancy and statutory bar).

Wherever possible, practices should endeavour to name a dismissal under one of these other four categories. SOSR should be used with caution and only after taking professional advice.

Claims of unfair dismissal

The five categories of potentially fair dismissal should enable an employer to establish a valid reason for a dismissal. If the employee feels he or she has been treated unfairly, then the determination of whether the dismissal was fair or unfair will be based on whether the employer acted reasonably or unreasonably in treating it as sufficient reason for dismissing the employee, taking into account the size and resources of the employer's organisation. That decision will be made by an employment tribunal or the new ACAS Unfair Dismissal Procedure. This new scheme can be used as an alternative to an employment tribunal and both are now described.

Employment tribunals

Employment tribunals were originally introduced to provide an informal and cheap method of settling disputes between individuals and their employers.

Tribunals are independent judicial bodies and their jurisdiction extends over England, Wales and Scotland. The country is divided into regions, each with their own regional chairman and regional office. Tribunals sit at various locations within their regions.

Employees who feel they have a claim for unfair dismissal against their employer must complete an IT1 form, giving the reasons why they are making a claim against the employer, and submit their application to the tribunal. This application must be made within three months of the dismissal taking place. The claim is registered by the tribunal, which sends a copy of the IT1 form to the employer with another form (IT3), which the employer completes and returns to the tribunal within 21 days. Form IT3 is the employer's response to the claim.

If the claim is not settled out of court or if the employee does not withdraw his or her claim, a hearing is held. Between the time the claim is registered and the date of the hearing, both parties prepare for the hearing, which these days usually includes hiring professional legal representation.

The hearing is held in public and the tribunal panel is normally comprised of three people – one representative from an employers' organisation, one representative from a trade union organisation and a chair, who will be legally qualified. Once the case is heard, with each party presenting their side, including witnesses who can be cross-examined, the hearing is adjourned for the tribunal to consider the evidence. The parties will be recalled to hear the decision of the tribunal and, if the employee wins the case, the re-engagement order (where the employer is instructed to re-employ the individual) or the compensation awarded.

Tribunals have become extremely formal, with both sides regularly employing legal professionals. They are also used far more frequently than first anticipated and are now a very costly and time-consuming apparatus for resolving industrial disputes.

The arbitration scheme

Description of the scheme

In recognition of the problems caused by the long delays and costs of employment tribunals, ACAS, under The Employment Rights (Dispute Resolution) Act 1998, has designed an arbitration scheme which echoes the very purpose for which employment tribunals were originally established. The aim of this new ACAS scheme is to provide parties with a more informal, private, quicker and cheaper method of resolving disputes.

Where parties to industrial disputes (including unfair dismissal) agree to put their disagreements to arbitration, the case can be heard by an independent arbitrator selected from an ACAS panel of persons with suitable industrial, academic and/or legal experience.

Use of the new scheme is voluntary and it can be used where conciliation has failed but both parties would like a decisive conclusion reached, as speedily as possible, with a minimum of formality and complete confidentiality. Once entered into, neither party can later take the claim to an employment tribunal or appeal against the arbitrator's decision, except in exceptional circumstances such as the clear incompetence or incapacity of the arbitrator.

Procedure at the hearing

Unlike tribunals, there is no requirement for oaths or affirmations. The process is inquisitorial rather than adversarial. Although witnesses are allowed and questions can be raised through the arbitrator, there is no cross-examination. Much emphasis is placed on both parties providing documentation relevant to their case, including forms IT1 and IT3. Documentation submitted is copied to the other party prior to the hearing.

After each side has presented their case, the arbitrator establishes the facts through questioning both parties. It is anticipated that most hearings will be completed within three or four hours.

The decision and award

The arbitrator considers carefully all the evidence, with reference to the ACAS Code of Practice on disciplinary procedures and the advisory booklet on discipline at work, rather than statute and case law.

About two weeks after the hearing, the decision is communicated to both parties and, if the dismissal is found to be unfair, the arbitrator may make a monetary award to the employee or order re-employment. Any compensation awarded is subject to the same limits as tribunal awards. The award is legally enforceable and the confidential property of both parties. There is no appeal.

The introduction of this new arbitration scheme is an attractive alternative to employment tribunals, particularly for smaller employers such as general practices, which do not have the resources to enter into complex and time-consuming tribunal proceedings. It is particularly appropriate for those employers and employees who wish to retain confidentiality and present their own case, without the need to be aware of legal precedent, in a forum which is non-adversarial and where the legal procedure is reduced to a minimum.

Conclusion

In conclusion, these two chapters focus on the end of the employment journey – terminating contracts of employment – and have provided guidelines and practical advice to primary healthcare organisations on the legal and effective management of terminating employment. These would stand scrutiny by a tribunal should practices find themselves subject to an allegation of unfair dismissal.

References

ACAS (1998) *Annual Report.* ACAS, London.

ACAS (2000) *Code of Practice on Disciplinary and Grievance Procedures in Employment.* HMSO, London

Chartered Institute of Personnel and Development (1997) *Employment Relations into the 21st Century. CIPD Position Paper.* CIPD, London.

Chief Medical Officer for England (1999) *Supporting Doctors, Protecting Patients.* HMSO, London

Commission for Racial Equality (1983) *Code of Practice for the Elimination of Racial Discrimination and the Promotion of Equality of Opportunity in Employment.* CRE, London.

Cooper C and Hoel H (2000) University of Manchester Institute of Science and Technology, Manchester.

Cunningham I (1994) *The Wisdom of Strategic Learning.* McGraw Hill, London.

Department of Education and Employment (1990) *Redundancy Payments.* HMSO, London.

Department of Education and Employment (1999a) *Equal Opportunities Ten Point Plan.* HMSO, London.

Department of Education and Employment (1999b) *Age Diversity in Employment (Code of Practice).* HMSO, London.

Department of Health (1997) *The New NHS: modern, dependable.* HMSO, London.

Department of Health (1998a) *Putting Patients First: the future of the NHS in Wales.* HMSO, London.

Department of Health (1998b) *Designed to Care: renewing the NHS in Scotland.* HMSO, London.

Department of Health (1998c) *A First Class Service: quality in the new NHS.* Health Service Circular HSC (98)113. HMSO, London.

Department of Trade and Industry (1999) *Employment Relations Act.* HMSO, London.

Elwyn G and Smail S (1998) *Personal and Practice Development Plans in Primary Care.* University of Wales College of Medicine, School of Postgraduate Medical and Dental Education, Cardiff.

Equal Opportunities Commission (1985) *Code of Practice for the Elimination of Discrimination on the Grounds of Sex and Marriage and the Promotion of Equality of Opportunity in Employment.* EOC, Manchester.

General Medical Council (2000) *Revalidating Doctors: ensuring standards, securing the future.* GMC, London.

Guest D and Conway N (1997) Employee motivation and the psychological contract. *People Management Magazine.* **3**(21).

Haman H and Irvine S (1998) Appraisal for general practice development: an evaluation of a programme of appraisal courses held in the Northern Region 1995–6. *Education for General Practice.* **9**(1): 44–50.

Hunt J (1990) *Managing People at Work* (2e). McGraw Hill, London.

Irvine D (1999) *The Performance of Doctors: quality, accountability and the public interest.* The Harben Lecture.

Irvine S and Haman H (1997) *Making Sense of Personnel Management* (2e). Radcliffe Medical Press, Oxford.

Irvine S and Haman H (2001) *Spotlight on General Practice: preparing for the demands of clinical governance and revalidation.* Radcliffe Medical Press. Oxford.

Marples S (1999) Learning to get ahead. *Health Management Magazine.* 24.

Midgley S (1999) Work of fiction. *People Management Magazine.* **5**(11): 58–60.

Prickett R (1998) *People Management Magazine.* **4**(21): 13.

Royal College of General Practitioners (1999) *An Initial Response to 'Supporting Doctors, Protecting Patients'*. RCGP, London.

Van Zwanenberg T and Harrison J (2000) *Clinical Governance in Primary Care*. Radcliffe Medical Press, Oxford.

Walsh J (1998) Staff in NHS stressed by bad practice. *People Management Magazine*. **4**(7): 13.

West M and Patterson M (1998) The Sheffield Effectiveness Programme. Institute of Work Psychology, University of Sheffield. *People Management Magazine*. **4**(1): 28–31.

Appendix A:
Sample equal opportunities policy for general practice

Anytown Surgery Equal Opportunities Policy

The practice policy

The practice is committed to a policy of equality of opportunity in its employment practices and in the provision of its services. It aims to ensure that no job applicant, employee, patient or any other person wishing to access and make use of its services receives less favourable treatment on the grounds of race (throughout this policy the word 'race' includes colour, nationality, ethnic and national origins), sex, sexual orientation, marital status or of other conditions not justified in law or relevant to the performance of the job. This applies to disabled people where the practice is able to offer suitable and safe employment to appropriately qualified applicants.

Individuals will be selected, promoted and treated on the basis of their abilities and merits, and according to the requirements of the job.

The responsibility for ensuring that the policy is implemented lies with the practice manager, who will report regularly on its implementation to the partners.

The scope of this policy

This policy applies to the partners and other health professionals who provide services to the practice's patients, and all practice employees.

The Equal Opportunities Policy and you

All partners and employees should be aware of the Equal Opportunities Policy and the obligations which fall on them to ensure its success and to comply with the provisions of the Acts.

You have a duty not to discriminate or to help others to do so. Compliance with these laws and the practice's policy is a personal responsibility for all employees. Incidents of sex/race or disability discrimination may be investigated in accordance with the terms of the disciplinary procedure.

If you consider that you are suffering from unequal treatment on the grounds of your sex, marital status, race, age or disability, you may make a complaint, which will be dealt with through the procedure for dealing with grievances as set out in the practice's grievance procedure.

If you consider that you are suffering from harassment on the grounds of race, religion, sex, sexual orientation, HIV/AIDS antibody status, age or disability, you may make a complaint under the practice's Harassment at Work Policy.

Legal background to the policy

It is the practice's policy to meet the provisions of the Sex Discrimination Act (SDA), the Equal Pay Act (EPA), the Race Relations Act (RRA) and the Disability Discrimination Act (DDA) which make it unlawful to discriminate on the grounds of sex, marital status, race and disability. The Rehabilitation of Offenders Act is also relevant. It may be helpful for all within the practice to have the following summary of these Acts.

The Sex Discrimination Act

This makes unlawful two kinds of discrimination on the grounds of sex and marriage. These are:

- *direct discrimination*, where a person treats a woman less favourably than he or she would a man on grounds of her sex, or a married person less favourably than an unmarried person of the same sex on the grounds of marital status. The Act also applies to a man who is treated less favourably than a woman
- *indirect discrimination*, where an unjustifiable requirement or condition is applied equally to both sexes, but has a disproportionately adverse effect on one sex because the proportion of one sex that can comply with it is considerably smaller than the proportion of the other sex. Some examples of indirect discrimination can be found below.

The Race Relations Act

This makes unlawful both direct and indirect discrimination on the grounds of colour, race, nationality, ethnic or national origins. Discrimination on grounds of religion is unlawful in Northern Ireland. The indirect discrimination clauses are broadly similar to those in the SDA described above.

Examples of indirect discrimination:

- applying an unjustifiable age barrier
- promoting according to seniority or 'buggin's turn'
- rigidly insisting on certain educational qualifications not essential to performance of the job
- selecting advertising media and/or publications to which sectors of society covered by the above Acts would not normally have access.

The Disability Discrimination Act

Knowledge of some of the detail of this Act is important as it is easy to discriminate unwittingly against people with disabilities.

This Act gives people with disabilities the right not to be discriminated against in employment as well as a right to access to goods and services.

Who is protected?

- job applicants
- employees
- apprentices
- people who contract personally to provide services.

The law covers people who are currently disabled as well as those who have had a disability in the past, including mental illness.

What is disability?

The Act defines it as a physical or mental impairment (mobility, manual dexterity, physical co-ordination, speech, hearing or eyesight), which has a substantial and long-term adverse effect on the person's ability to carry out normal day-to-day activities.

Mental impairment includes only those resulting from clinically well-recognised illnesses, while 'long-term effects' are those which have lasted at least 12 months or can reasonably be expected to last at least that long.

Severe disfigurement is seen as having a substantial adverse effect and therefore comes within the scope of the Act if it is an impairment that is controlled or corrected by, for example, medication, artificial limbs or hearing aids. However, sight impairment that can be corrected by spectacles or contact lenses is outside the scope of the Act.

Progressive conditions such as HIV infection, cancer and multiple sclerosis are regarded as disabilities even before they have had a substantial effect on normal day-to-day activities, as long as the condition is ultimately expected to result in such an effect.

What does it cover?

Where a disabled person applies for a job or makes inquiries about it, the employer must not discriminate:

- in the recruitment and selection process
- in the terms and conditions on which that individual is offered a job.

Where a disabled person is in employment, the employer must not discriminate on grounds related to his or her disability:

- in the terms of employment
- in the opportunities for promotion, transfer, training or other benefits
- by dismissing him or her.

The Act also requires employers to make 'reasonable adjustment' to working arrangements or the workplace where that would have overcome the practical effects of a disability.

The Rehabilitation of Offenders Act

This Act prohibits recruiters from asking about convictions which are spent (except in certain exempted professions). An applicant is entitled to deny that he or she has a criminal record if the conviction(s) are spent.

Recruitment procedures

It is at the point of recruitment and selection that most illegal discrimination takes place. It is all too easy to recruit people who reflect ourselves in terms of colour, class, age, etc. To ensure that the practice attracts and keeps the best people, the practice's recruitment procedure, as described below, must be followed.

The principles of the recruitment and selection procedure are as follows:

- all personnel who are involved in the recruitment and selection of staff should be familiar with the main principles of the above legislation, and fundamental to compliance is the adoption of procedures and techniques, including questioning techniques, which serve to eradicate unlawful direct and indirect discrimination
- job descriptions are clearly and concisely written and free from illegal bias
- personal specifications only detail criteria relevant to the performance of the job
- advertisements are free from unlawful discrimination in both words and pictures and state that the practice aims to be an equal opportunities employer
- all vacancies are advertised both internally and externally. A vacant post will be advertised internally only where exceptional circumstances prevail, including knowledge of the market and unavailability of suitable external candidates. It is anticipated that lateral transfers and promotions involving minor changes to the post-holder's sphere of responsibility would be excluded from this requirement to advertise externally
- agencies which may be involved in the recruitment process, e.g. temporary staff agencies and recruitment consultants, are informed of and given a copy of this policy

- all recruitment interviews require the presence of a senior member of staff or partner who has received equal opportunities training in the recruitment and selection of staff
- at no time during the recruitment process should applicants be asked inappropriate or illegal questions
- clear records of the reasons for decisions made throughout the recruitment process should be maintained as should notes of each interview, which should include the questions asked of each candidate.

The job description and personal specification

These documents are crucial in ensuring that as objective an assessment as possible is used in selecting the right candidate. The job description describes the main duties and responsibilities of the vacancy and must be written before the personal specification, which describes the type of person needed to undertake those duties and responsibilities.

It is easy to merge the two and immediately start imagining the type of person to employ before a complete analysis and description of the post has taken place.

The personal specification is the document that translates the job description into a profile of the person required to do the job. This profile is expressed in terms of the qualities needed and whether such qualities are essential or merely desirable.

Applications

Applications need to be screened according to the personal specification. This is where the time and effort invested in designing and preparing this document reap huge benefits in terms of objectivity and time and, crucially, ensuring that the practice does not illegally discriminate against applicants. This system of shortlisting for interview ensures that only objective and lawful criteria are being used in the selection process, thereby minimising the risks of prejudice and subjectivity.

The interview

At interview, areas to explore need to have been allocated and each interviewer should write down the opening and follow-up questions in his or her area of questioning. All questions should relate to the qualities sought as identified on the personal specification and should not, under any circumstances, stray into such discriminatory areas as childcare arrangements, family planning intentions, etc.

To help the interview, a record will be kept of each candidate's response, by way of the practice's recruitment assessment form. The assessment form is used to:

- minimise the problem of interviewers confusing the candidates
- ensure a record is being maintained throughout the interview
- help identify discrepancies which can be explored later in the interview
- is in accordance with the ACAS Codes of Practice on the elimination of sex and race discrimination in employment
- help ensure that assessments made about a candidate are objective.

Selecting the successful candidate

Selecting the successful candidate is done only after all candidates have been interviewed and each has been assessed in relation to the job description and personal specification. The interview assessment form is extremely useful at this point in the process. It provides the objective record of the candidate's history and interview performance against which the personal specification is compared. The temptation, at this point, to compare candidates with each other must be resisted; if it is not, the best candidate may be appointed but the best may be the best of a bad or mediocre bunch and not the right candidate for the job.

Documentation

The recruitment and selection of staff should be carefully documented. Accurate notes and the reasons for selecting and rejecting at each stage should be maintained. There are two main reasons for keeping such documentation. The first relates to applicants' rights under data protection legislation to have access to personal data. The second reason relates to circumstances where illegal discrimination is alleged. Such records would play a crucial role in the practice's defence should it be sued for illegal discrimination. Indeed, not to have maintained such records would be viewed as a breach of the ACAS Codes of Practice in this area of employment law.

Training and promotion

No member of staff will be treated less favourably on the above defined grounds for the purposes of selection for training or promotion. The induction training of new staff will include training in this policy.

Age discrimination

There is no law against discriminating on grounds of age other than if it constitutes indirect unlawful discrimination. The practice has a retirement age of ..., and below this age will ensure that unless there is a relevant reason, there will be no automatic exclusion of entire age groups from employment opportunities.

As a general rule, age will not be used as a primary discriminator in recruitment, selection, promotion and training decisions.

Appendix B:
Sample prevention of harassment policy for general practice

Anytown Surgery – Prevention of Harassment Policy

The practice policy

The practice has drawn up a policy to help prevent harassment and deal with allegations of harassment if they occur.

The practice is committed to equality of opportunity in employment and believes that all employees should be treated with respect and dignity in the workplace and in the course of their work. Harassment on the grounds of race, religion, sex, sexual orientation, HIV/AIDS antibody status, age or disability, will not be tolerated and proven complaints will be dealt with under the provisions of this policy, which can include the practice's disciplinary procedure.

This document provides advice and guidance on dealing with harassment. It:

- is compliant with UK legislation
- defines harassment and identifies examples of such behaviour and the forms it can take
- identifies the responsibilities of partners, managers and employees in creating an atmosphere where equality flourishes and where harassment is not tolerated

- clarifies that complaints of harassment should be dealt with through the disciplinary procedure.

The scope of this policy

This policy applies to all members of the primary healthcare team, including temporary staff.

Employees will be expected to follow this policy in their dealings with patients and other people from outside the practice. It is not possible to apply the provisions in this document to service users or suppliers who are not employees of the practice. It may be possible to counter harassment in other ways and the partners will give support in whatever way is appropriate to any employee who is harassed in the course of his or her work by someone who is not a practice employee. Any allegations of harassment by a partner will be dealt with by the other members of the partnership.

The legal background to the policy

Racial harassment can constitute unlawful racial discrimination under the Race Relations Act 1976.

Sexual harassment can constitute unlawful sex discrimination under the Sex Discrimination Act 1975 and the EC Resolution (December 1991) extends to sex-based conduct and includes verbal and non-verbal as well as physical conduct.

Bullying and intimidatory behaviour can constitute intentional harassment under the Criminal Justice and Public Order Act 1994.

Definition of harassment

Harassment is unacceptable behaviour towards an individual that is based on that individual's race, religion, sex, sexual orientation, HIV/AIDS antibody status, age or disability and which is unreasonable, unwelcome or offensive.

It also includes harassment, bullying and intimidatory behaviour based on factors (often unknown) other than those detailed above.

Harassment affects the dignity of men and women at work. Harassment will normally be a pattern of behaviour which continues over a period of time and which is unwanted, unreciprocated and uninvited by the recipient. However, an isolated incident or incidents over a short period of time can also constitute harassment.

Examples of behaviour which may constitute harassment include the following:

- *physical harassment*: unwanted touching or petting, pinching or unnecessarily brushing against someone, physical assault and enforced sexual attention
- *verbal harassment*: persistent name calling, sexual propositioning, making offensive comments or jokes about a person based on his or her race, religion, sex, sexual orientation, HIV/AIDS antibody status, age or disability
- *non-verbal harassment*: displaying posters or material, writing graffiti that is sexist or racist, anti-gay or anti-lesbian or offensive to disabled people. Displaying emblems, symbols and flags which may be offensive to particular religious or other ethnic/national groups
- *bullying*: a pattern of intimidatory behaviour which can be both verbal and non-verbal.

If the perpetrator of any of the above adopts behaviour of non-co-operation or abuses his or her position in relation to the person who alleges harassment (e.g. withholding information, sabotaging work, discriminating in the areas of promotion and training opportunities), this too will constitute harassment.

This list is not intended to be exhaustive. There may be more subtle behaviour, which will be perceived by the recipient as harassment.

Partners' and managers' responsibility

Partners and managers have an essential role in implementing this policy, not only in dealing promptly with complaints of harassment but in creating an environment where harassment is not tolerated and where all individuals are treated with respect and dignity.

Partners and managers are responsible for setting examples and standards of behaviour in the workplace and to ensure that the staff they manage are aware of the details of this policy.

Managers, and particularly the partner responsible for staff, will be responsible for providing support for those individuals they manage who are suffering harassment, for helping stop harassment, for being alert to any such incidents and for intervening appropriately and promptly.

Employees' responsibility

Employees are responsible for adhering to this policy. They are required to treat work colleagues with respect and dignity, not to condone harassment and to bring any such behaviour to the attention of the practice manager, the partner responsible for staff or any other partner they choose as appropriate in line with the complaints procedure below.

Complaints

An investigation into allegations of harassment can prove traumatic and stressful for all parties and it is essential that the matter is handled quickly and in a sensitive and tactful manner.

It is helpful and preferable, in most cases, for the matter to be dealt with informally.

The employee should make a note of the details of the harassment, which will be important should a formal complaint be made later. The following information should be recorded:

- date of first and subsequent incidents of harassment
- location of incident
- nature of incident (to cover both actions and comments of the other party or parties)
- feelings of the person being harassed at the time
- names of any witnesses.

This information should be kept safely until the matter has been resolved.

An alleged harasser may be unaware that their behaviour is causing discomfort or offence and may stop if informed of its impact. It is important therefore that, as soon as possible after the harassment starts, the employee should make it clear that he or she finds the behaviour uncomfortable and/or offensive. Even the most confident of people find confronting unacceptable behaviour in others difficult. However, as a first step, discussing the behaviour with the alleged harasser can stop the behaviour and prevent the issue from escalating.

If the harassment is by a supervisor, manager or partner, then the employee can seek support from the manager/partner of his or her choice.

The complainant may sometimes find it difficult to make it clear to the alleged harasser that the behaviour is offensive and in those circumstances he or she should enlist the support of the appropriate manager or partner of their choice.

All discussions at this stage will be confidential and informal. Notes of the complaint will be taken by the manager/partner and the possible options for dealing with the situation will be discussed.

In all cases where the complainant has not been able to stop the harassment, for whatever reason, including a reluctance to approach the harasser direct, and has notified management of the harassment, the manager/partner will discuss the complaint with the partner responsible for staff and determine the most appropriate method of dealing with the matter.

The severity of the complaint, both in terms of incidents and frequency, will determine the most appropriate option of dealing with the matter. Options can include the partner responsible for staff, with the practice manager (if appropriate) promptly and impartially investigating the facts with due regard to the rights of both parties. Depending on the outcome of this investigation, either one may speak to the alleged harasser to seek resolution. This may be as simple as gaining an assurance from the alleged harasser that there will be no recurrence or clarifying the reasons for the behaviour and whether there is an explanation which can be accepted by the complainant.

Where such an assurance is later broken, or in cases of serious harassment, the matter will be reported to the partnership. They will determine the most appropriate partner to invoke the practice's disciplinary procedure. This includes a thorough investigation of the facts and a disciplinary hearing where the alleged harasser will have the full opportunity to state his or her case.

Throughout both informal and, where practicable, formal investigations and resolutions, the confidentiality of all involved, including witnesses, will be maintained.

Malicious complaints are rare; where they do occur they will be dealt with under the disciplinary procedure.

After the procedure

Where a complaint is upheld it may be necessary to consider transferring one party. Given the relatively small size of the practice, transfers may not always be practicable. However, where practicable, the complainant should be given first choice whether he or she wishes to be transferred. Where a transfer occurs, it will not lead to any disadvantage for the complainant.

If a complaint is not upheld, consideration may still be given, again wherever practicable, to the voluntary transfer of one of the employees concerned. This is preferable to requiring them to continue to work together against the wishes of either party.

Support and counselling

The practice is not equipped to provide specialist counselling internally. The role of the practice manager and the partner responsible for staff, as with other managers and partners, is to provide support which may include referring either party to outside counsellors. As harassment cases may involve disciplinary action, undertaking a professional counselling role in such cases would be inappropriate.

Where a complaint has been upheld, both through the informal and/or formal procedure, it is important for the practice's manager and whichever partner has been involved to check that harassment has stopped and that there has been no victimisation. Careful monitoring will be undertaken, which may involve a number of methods, including observing behaviour and interviewing the complainant.

Appendix C:
Individual rights arising
from employment

This list is not exhaustive but it does cover the major statutory employment rights of employees. There are exceptions to eligibility to many of these rights, which are not appropriate to list here. This list is a general guide only.

Rights needing a qualifying period of continuous employment

Rights	Service
Minimum period of notice	one month
Guarantee payment	one month
Pay during suspension on medical grounds	one month*
Not to be unfairly dismissed	one year
Redundancy payment	two years
Time off to seek alternative work or arrange training in a redundancy situation	two years
In a redundancy situation, to a trial period where alternative employment is offered, without forfeiting right to redundancy payment	two years
Additional maternity leave	one year
Parental leave	one year

* Except when related to pregnancy or maternity, in which case there is no qualifying period.

Rights of all employees regardless of length of service

- Access to medical reports provided by a medical practitioner for employment purposes.
- To conceal past convictions where the conviction has become spent (exceptions include medical practitioners, nurses, midwives and any profession to which the Supplementary to the Medicine Act 1960 applies and which is undertaken following registration under that Act).
- Not to be discriminated against on grounds of disability (unless the reason can be justified).
- Not to be discriminated against on grounds of sex, parental or marital status.
- Not to be discriminated against on racial grounds.
- Not to be discriminated against on grounds of part-time status.
- Not to be victimised for taking part in trade union activities.
- Not to be victimised for whistle blowing.
- To time off for antenatal care.
- To basic maternity leave.
- To statutory maternity pay.
- To return to work after absence on maternity leave.
- To time off for dependants.
- To remuneration under a protective award.
- To statements of terms and conditions of employment (to be given to employees within their first two months of service).
- To receive a minimum wage.
- To be given an itemised pay statement.
- Not to have deductions made from salaries unless contractually agreed or required by statute.
- To four weeks' annual holiday with pay.
- To work no more than 48 hours per week with appropriate rest periods for night workers.
- To take time off for public duties.

- To time off as an official of a recognised independent trade union.
- To time off to take part in activities of an independent recognised trade union.
- To time off to perform the functions of a safety representative.
- Not to be dismissed for a pregnancy or maternity-related reason.
- Not to be dismissed for drawing attention to a health and safety matter.
- Not to be dismissed for asserting a statutory right.
- Not to be dismissed for any reason connected with membership of an independent trade union.
- To representation at a serious disciplinary or grievance hearing.

Appendix D:
Sample disciplinary procedure for general practice

Anytown Surgery – Disciplinary Procedure

These disciplinary rules and procedures have been set up to promote fairness in the treatment of individuals, so that members of staff know the standards of work and conduct expected of them. The procedure should ensure that these standards are maintained and also provide a fair method of dealing with alleged failures to observe these standards.

The rules and procedures are intended to uphold standards of work and conduct and where necessary to improve them. They ensure that all staff are entitled to:

- fair and consistent treatment
- assistance with improving standards which are below acceptable levels
- adequate warning and speedy consideration of any disciplinary matter
- appeal procedures against decisions about disciplinary matters
- the right to be accompanied.

Definitions

Misconduct

- Minor breaches of discipline such as:
    - poor attendance and time keeping
    - refusal to obey reasonable instructions
    - minor insubordination
    - minor infringements of the practice's Health and Safety at Work Policy (this list is not exhaustive).
- Serious misconduct; while the following list is not exhaustive (nor intended to be) this may be taken to include:
    - unauthorised removal of the practice's property
    - minor breach of confidentiality
    - neglect of duties
    - illegal act of sex, race or disability discrimination
    - breach of the practice's Health and Safety Policy, Harassment at Work Policy or Equal Opportunities Policy
    - persistent minor breaches of discipline
    - persistent failure to achieve agreed standards of conduct
    - flagrant failure to follow documented procedures and regulations
    - working for another employer without the prior express agreement of the practice
    - behaviour outside work which is likely to have an adverse effect on the practice's reputation or if the behaviour makes the employee unsuitable for his/her position.
- Gross misconduct; conduct of a nature serious enough to justify summary dismissal. While the following list is not exhaustive (nor intended to be) this may be taken to include:
    - dishonesty or behaviour of a grossly unseemly nature in the course of employment, or private life, if the behaviour is likely to have an adverse effect on the reputation of the practice or makes the member of staff unsuitable to hold his/her position
    - serious breach of confidentiality

- gross neglect of duties
- serious breach of sex, race or disability discrimination Acts
- any wilful or serious breach of the practice's Health and Safety Policy, Harassment at Work Policy or Equal Opportunities Policy
- abuse of drugs
- being under the influence of drink or drugs during working hours
- aggressive behaviour in the workplace or gross insubordination
- falsification of the practice's administrative records
- misuse, or use for personal gain, of equipment or information belonging to the practice
- forgery or fraud
- any other misdeed which might warrant suspension or dismissal, including repeated or persistent minor breaches of discipline.

Disciplinary action

The following action can be taken by the practice:

- to issue a warning to the employee with details of the consequences of any further breaches of discipline
- transfer – a change of job. If the new job is of a lower grade than the present position, the salary and benefits levels will be those of the lower grade
- dismissal – termination by the practice of the employee's contract of employment with due notice
- summary dismissal – termination by the practice of the employee's contract of employment without notice.

The disciplinary procedures – misconduct

Any disciplinary action to be taken will be reasonable, taking into account the employee's record and any other relevant factors.

Preliminary procedure

In the normal course of events individual members of staff may be warned about faults in their conduct. Such preliminary warnings will not form part of the disciplinary procedure and will normally be issued by the practice manager. At this stage it is expected that every effort will be made to train, guide or help the employee to bring his or her conduct to an acceptable standard within an agreed timescale. If assistance is given to an employee to achieve the improvement required, this information will be noted on the employee's file and a copy of the note given to them.

When the above actions are either not appropriate or proving unsuccessful, the formal procedure, as set out below, should be implemented:

Stage 1. Misconduct: formal warning

In the case of misconduct, the individual should be given a formal verbal warning or, if the circumstances are more serious, a written warning, setting out the nature of the breach of conduct and the action that will be taken if further breaches occur.

The individual will also be advised that the warning constitutes the first stage of the formal disciplinary procedure, the conduct that is required and the timescale during which an improvement will be expected. The warning will be recorded on the individual's file.

Written warnings and more serious disciplinary action can only be taken by the partners, excluding the partner who is responsible for receiving appeals against disciplinary action taken.

Stage 2. Misconduct: final warning

Serious misconduct or further breaches of conduct which have occasioned a previous warning will lead to a final written warning being issued. The warning will specify the action which will be taken in the event of a repetition of the breach of conduct. The action taken can be either dismissal with notice, transfer or suspension without pay as appropriate. Timescales for improvement, where appropriate, will be specified.

Stage 3. Misconduct: dismissal or transfer

Failure to improve after a final warning or conduct regarded as gross misconduct, will lead to dismissal or transfer to another job, depending on the nature of the misconduct.

Any decision to dismiss or transfer can only be taken by the partners, excluding the partner responsible for hearing appeals against the disciplinary action taken.

Gross misconduct

In the event of any alleged serious or gross misconduct, an enquiry will be conducted and a full investigation will take place. This enquiry will be undertaken by the practice manager and/or one of the partners, as appropriate in the circumstances. Following the enquiry and investigations the following actions, appropriate to the circumstances, may be taken:

- take no further action, issue a verbal warning or issue a formal written warning
- dismiss (either with or without notice as may be appropriate)
- take such other disciplinary steps (e.g. transfer or demotion) as may be appropriate.

General points

Generally in connection with disciplinary procedures.

- At any interview or meeting at any stage in the disciplinary procedure the member of staff will be given a full opportunity to explain or state her or his case.
- In any disciplinary interview or hearing which may result in a formal warning or other serious action, the employee has the right to be accompanied by a representative. If a member of a trade union, the employee may be accompanied by his or her trade union representative. If not a member of a trade union the employee may be accompanied by a fellow employee of his or her choice.
- The representative will be able to address the hearing and confer with the employee but they will not be able to answer questions on behalf of the employee.
- The hearing will be postponed up to a maximum of five working days if the employee's chosen representative is not available on the first occasion.
- In appropriate circumstances, the practice may suspend an employee from duty with pay for the purpose of the investigation of a complaint.
- Where a written warning is given, the member of staff may be required to sign an acknowledgement of receipt.
- A copy of any written warning will be retained in the member of staff's personnel file. The length of time during which any warning remains effective will vary depending on the circumstances. They will be informed of the length of time applicable to any specific warning. Only in exceptional circumstances will a warning remain effective for more than one year.
- Formal disciplinary interviews will be chaired by a partner with another partner and/or the practice manager in attendance. A record of the interview will be produced within 48 hours and agreed with both parties.
- The employee may appeal against any disciplinary action taken against him or her. The appeal should be made in writing to Dr ...... unless he or she has been involved in the disciplinary decision, then the appeal should be made to

Dr . . . . Any such appeal should be put in writing stating the grounds of the appeal and made within five working days of receipt of the warning or dismissal.

- The full disciplinary procedure is not intended to apply to a member of staff during his or her probationary period, during which time any measures taken and procedures adopted shall be wholly at the discretion of the partners.

- The practice's disciplinary procedure applies to the practice manager. However, authority to conduct a disciplinary inquiry, warning or dismissal can only be taken by Drs . . . . . . and . . . .

The disciplinary procedure – unsatisfactory performance

Consistently poor performance of duties is usually a result of either misconduct or incapability. If poor performance is a matter of misconduct, then the disciplinary procedures will be followed. However, if incapability is an issue, the stages followed, although similar to those of the disciplinary procedure, are designed to provide the member of staff concerned with structured support and help to improve his or her performance. Should an improvement in performance not be achieved, the above stages will be used as a guide to any ultimate dismissal.

Appendix E:
Sample grievance procedure for general practice

Anytown Surgery – Grievance Procedure

Any grievance you may have which relates to your employment and which cannot be resolved informally should be raised through the following procedure.

Stage 1

The employee shall, in the first instance, discuss the grievance with his or her line manager, who will be either [*job title*] or the practice manager, who will investigate and report back to the employee within seven working days, where practicable.

If the grievance involves the line manager, then the employee should omit Stage 1 and go straight to Stage 2.

Stage 2

Failing a satisfactory solution under Stage 1, the employee should detail the grievance in writing, which should be given to the partner responsible for staff. A copy should also be given to their immediate line manager. The partner will investigate the grievance and report back, both verbally and in writing, to the employee within seven working days, where practicable, of receipt of the written grievance.

Stage 3

Failing a resolution under Stage 2, the employee will make a written submission to the partnership, who will investigate the grievance and report back, both verbally and in writing, to the employee within two weeks, where practicable, of receipt of the written submission.

The Partnership's decision on the grievance is final.

Under Stages 2 and 3, where interviewing the employee forms part of the investigation, the employee will have the right to be accompanied by a representative. If a member of a trade union, the employee may be accompanied by his or her trade union representative. If not a member of a trade union, the employee may be accompanied by a fellow employee of his or her choice.

The representative will be able to address the partner/partnership (as appropriate) conducting the interview and confer with the employee, but they will not be able to answer questions on behalf of the employee.

The hearing will be postponed up to a maximum of five working days if the employee's chosen representative is not available on the first occasion.

Appendix F:
Principles of the ACAS Code of Practice on disciplinary procedures in employment (May 2000)

- **Be in writing**. The disciplinary rules and procedure should be written clearly and be available to all employees.
- **Specify to whom they apply**. If particular rules or procedures only apply to a certain category of staff then this should be made clear. The usual exception to procedures are probationary staff.
- **Be non-discriminatory**. The rules should be applied consistently and fairly, ensuring that neither the disciplinary rules themselves nor their application discriminates against any employee on the basis of their sex, marital status, race, disability and any other category of illegal discrimination.
- **Provide for matters to be dealt with without undue delay**. The procedure should be designed to allow enough time for the disciplinary issue to be thoroughly investigated without taking so much time that the employee is caused undue stress.
- **Provide for proceedings, witness statements and records to be kept confidential**. To ensure that only those directly involved in the disciplinary issue are allowed access to the proceedings and above identified documents.

- **Indicate the disciplinary actions which may be taken**. In addition to the obvious actions – verbal, written, final written warnings and dismissal – any alternatives to dismissal should be specified. If a practice decides to suspend without pay or demote as forms of disciplinary action, these must be specified in order to protect the organisation against a civil court action for breach of contract.
- **Specify the levels of management that have authority to take the various forms of disciplinary action and ensure that immediate superiors do not normally have the power to dismiss without reference to senior management**. In a practice this will probably be written, as the practice manager has the authority to issue verbal (or even written) warnings to all ancillary staff, but any decision to dismiss can only be taken by a partner. Allowing the practice manager authority to dismiss would be in contravention of this guideline.
- **Provide for individuals to be informed of the complaints against them and where possible all relevant evidence before any hearing**. The complaint(s) should be detailed in writing and accompanied by copies of the evidence which will be produced at the disciplinary hearing.
- **Provide employees with an opportunity to state their case before decisions are reached**. Enough time should elapse between receipt of the letter informing them of the allegations (and any evidence) and the interview to allow the employee to marshal any evidence *they* may wish to present in their defence. It is important to allow employers, during the disciplinary hearing, to state their case, including any mitigating circumstances, before any disciplinary decision is made.
- **Give individuals the right to be accompanied by a trade union representative or, if not a member of a trade union, by a fellow employee of their choice**. Appendix D and Chapter 5 detail an employee's rights to be accompanied.

- **Ensure that, except for gross misconduct, no employee is dismissed for a first breach of discipline**. Although employers are free to design their own disciplinary rules, a practice which dismisses for a first breach of time-keeping rules, for example, would be in contravention of this guideline. Examples of what constitutes gross misconduct should be specified in the rules.
- **Ensure that disciplinary action is not taken until the case has been carefully investigated**. Thorough investigation is crucial to handling a disciplinary issue fairly. Even the most clear-cut breaches need careful examination. Second-hand information and hearsay are not acceptable. It is important to take a written record of the investigation because if facing a tribunal, comprehensive and detailed notes of the investigation may be crucial to the case.
- **Ensure that individuals are given an explanation for any penalty imposed**. Such explanations should be given verbally in a meeting and then confirmed in writing. A verbal warning need not be confirmed in the form of a letter – a record of the disciplinary interview and any subsequent meeting can instead be given to the employee.
- **Provide a right of appeal and specify the procedure to be followed**. The employee should be informed verbally of the above and this should be confirmed in writing. It is usual for the written warning letter or dismissal letter to explain the appeal procedure in the final paragraph.

Index